The Diabetic **CHOCOLATE** COOKBOOK

—

MARY JANE FINSAND

—

Foreword by James D. Healy, M.D., F.A.A.P.

Sterling Publishing Co., Inc.   New York

Edited and designed by Vilma Liacouras Chantiles

Library of Congress Cataloging in Publication Data

Finsand, Mary Jane.
  The diabetic chocolate cookbook.

  Includes index.
  1. Diabetes—Diet therapy—Recipes. 2. Cookery
(Chocolate) I. Title.
RC662.F565   1984   641.6'374   84-8454
ISBN 0-8069-5580-5
ISBN 0-8069-7900-3 (pbk.)

Copyright © 1984 by Mary Jane Finsand
Published by Sterling Publishing Co., Inc.
387 Park Avenue South, New York, N.Y. 10016
Distributed in Canada by Sterling Publishing
℅ Canadian Manda Group, P.O. Box 920, Station U
Toronto, Ontario, Canada M8Z 5P9
Distributed in Great Britain and Europe by Cassell PLC
Artillery House, Artillery Row, London SW1P 1RT, England
Distributed in Australia by Capricorn Ltd.
P.O. Box 665, Lane Cove, NSW 2066
Manufactured in the United States of America

Contents

Appendix • 141

Foreword

Chocolate is a favorite flavor throughout the world. But, chocolate is usually used to flavor highly sweetened foods such as candies and desserts. In the past, diabetics and others who needed to plan their diet were not allowed the luxury of eating chocolate foods because of the high energy sucrose that they contained.

Because a diet is the actual food we eat, everyone is "on a diet" whether the diet is planned or accidental. Even persons on accidental unlimited diets tend to consume excessive amounts of sugar in the foods they eat. Weight dieters, diabetics, persons on medically prescribed diets and almost everyone could benefit by reducing the amount of sucrose in their chocolate foods by using the recipes in Mary Jane Finsand's *The Diabetic Chocolate Cookbook.*

Each recipe is complete with calories and food exchange information to allow users to regulate food intake within medically prescribed doctor recommendations.

I believe that this cookbook will be a very usable kitchen reference for preparing sweet-tasting chocolate foods that have a minimum of sucrose and calories. Mary Jane has created another medically sound book to complement her previous books, *The Complete Diabetic Cookbook* and *Diabetic Candy, Cookie & Dessert Cookbook.*

James D. Healy, M.D., F.A.A.P.

A Recommendation from Schoitz Medical Center

Diabetic cookbooks usually say, "Never eat chocolate candy," especially to individuals on a controlled meal plan.

Now with the assistance of Mary Jane Finsand's *The Diabetic Chocolate Cookbook*, it is possible. This cookbook lists the food exchanges and, with carefully planned menus, chocolate candies may be included. We recommend an assortment of cookbooks for a variety of reasons and Mrs. Finsand's cookbook is among these. It is very easy to read; secondly, it reviews the sugar substitutes and food exchanges for the diabetic and other weight-conscious individuals.

Basic baking techniques in most of the recipes are easy enough for experienced teenagers to prepare with little or no supervision. In our opinion, this cookbook will be helpful, not only to the diabetic or weight-conscious person, but to the entire family, minimizing the hassle in food preparation.

Darlene Duke, R.N.
Hattie Middleton, R.D.
Schoitz Diabetes Education Resource Center
Schoitz Medical Center

Introduction

OH, YOU CHOCOLATE LOVERS! How old were you when you first tasted sweet, delicious chocolate and fell in love with it? Like love, chocolate is always a delight to receive or to give. We all know any chocolate dessert or snack will be considered a treat and a luxury. You, as a diabetic or weight-conscious individual, know better than anyone else, for you have had to remove most chocolate products "out" of your diet.

Now with new knowledge of the sugar substitutes and careful cooking, you can bring chocolate back into your diet as a luxury. *But only as a luxury.* It is impossible for you to have chocolate every day, and you know it. But you can allow yourself a little freedom within your diet, as long as you know the exchange values and calorie count of your foods.

As I did with *The Complete Diabetic Cookbook* and the *Diabetic Candy, Cookie & Dessert Cookbook*, I will help remove the word "restricted" from your eating. And so, I ask you to promise not to cheat on your diet. For this promise, I will create a little chocolate magic and a sense of perfection for your eating pleasure. I give you *The Diabetic Chocolate Cookbook* with my affection.

Mary Jane Finsand

Sugar and Sugar Replacements and Your Diet

Your diet has been prescribed by a doctor or diet counsellor who has been trained to determine your diet requirements by considering your daily life-style of exercise and calorie needs. *Do not* try to out-guess them. Always stay within the guidelines of your individual diet and ask your counsellor about additions or substitutions in your diet. If you have any questions about any diabetic recipes or exchanges, ask your diet counsellor.

There have been reports stating that diabetics could eat table sugar, such as sugars made from cane or beets. The research found that refined sugar did not get into the blood any more quickly than does sugar from wheat flour or potatoes. These reports contend that because all these products are starches, they could be eaten at meal-time. Because diabetics *MUST* keep the numbers of calories constant in their diets, they are usually told to avoid products containing sugar.

Sugar has approximately 770 calories per cup with 199 grams of carbohydrates; refined wheat flour has approximately 420 calories per cup with 88 grams of carbohydrates and the remaining calories are made up from the 12 grams of protein. Therefore, you would have to eat 2.26 times the amount of wheat flour to gain the same amount of grams of carbohydrates from one cup of sugar. By using one of the sugar replacements or new natural sweeteners on the market, you cut out most of the carbohydrates and calories normally gained when using a cane or beet sugar.

Now, let's put this fact into a food product. Say we make a basic chocolate cake with sugar and the very same chocolate cake with one of the sugar replacements, and this cake takes one cup of sugar. In the total cake with the sugar replacement, we have reduced the calories by approximately 770. That is a lot of calories and adds up to a lot of exchange values. If we sweeten a single cup of coffee or tea with two teaspoons of sugar, we add 30 calories (¾ Fruit Exchange), but if we sweeten it with an aspartame product we gain only four calories and with a sugar substitute we gain approximately two to three calories. Now those are major differences in calorie counts.

Most sweeteners or sugar replacements can be found in your super-market. They vary in sweetness, aftertaste, aroma and calories. The listing below is by ingredient name rather than product name. Check the side of the box or bottle to determine the contents of the product.

Aspartame and aspartame products are fairly new to the super-market. Aspartame is a natural protein sweetener; it is not an ar-tificial sweetener. Because of its intense sweetness, it reduces calories and carbohydrates in the diet. Aspartame has no aftertaste and a sweet aroma but loses part of its sweetness in heating. It does seem to complement some of the other sweeteners by removing their bitter aftertaste, however. Aspartame is recommended for use in cold prod-ucts.

Cyclamates and products containing cyclamates are less intense as sweeteners than the saccharin products; but they also leave a bitter aftertaste. Many of our sugar replacements are a combination of sac-charin and cyclamates.

Fructose or *levulose* is commonly known as fruit sugar. It is a natu-rally occurring sugar found in fruits and honey. The taste of fruit sugar (fructose) is the same as that of common table sugar (sucrose). But because of its intense sweetness, you use less fructose and thus reduce calories and carbohydrates in the diet. Fructose is not affected by heating or cooling and tends to add moisture to baked products.

Glycyrrhizin and products containing glycyrrhizin are sweeteners as intense as saccharin. They are seen less in supermarkets, because they give the food products a licorice taste and aroma.

Granular or dry sugar replacements containing sodium saccharin give less aftertaste to foods that are heated.

Liquid sugar replacements containing sodium saccharin are best used in cold foods or added to the food after it has partially cooled and no longer needs any heating.

Saccharin and products containing saccharin are the most widely known and used of the intense sweeteners. When used in baking or cooking, saccharin has a bitter, lingering aftertaste. You will nor-mally find it in the form of sodium saccharin in products labelled low-calorie sugar replacements. These include liquid and granulated brown sugar replacements used in this book.

Sorbitol is used in many of our commercial food products. It has little or no aftertaste and has a sweet aroma. At present, it can only be bought in bulk form at health food stores.

Chocolate Products, Carob and Imitation Chocolate

Baking cocoa is unsweetened chocolate with some of the cocoa butter removed and then powdered.

Baking or unsweetened chocolate is a pure chocolate which is moulded into blocks. It is the most commonly used chocolate in baking and cooking.

Carob is not a chocolate product. People with chocolate allergies, however, can use carob and still get the chocolate flavor. Many people prefer the carob flavor to chocolate; others notice a distinct difference between the two flavors. Although many people think there is a wide calorie count difference between carob and chocolate products, one tablespoon of carob has the **same** calorie count as one tablespoon of cocoa. And in most carob candy products, the calorie count will equal that of a comparable chocolate product because of the addition of extra fat. Therefore, if you have an allergy to chocolate, you may use equal amounts of a carob product for any chocolate product in the recipes in this book.

Dietetic dipping or coating chocolate is a special chocolate or chocolate-flavored product formulated to reduce calories in a candy product. For this reason it is the only dipping chocolate used in this book. I developed a Semisweet Dipping Chocolate recipe (page 16), used in many recipes in this book.

German chocolate is semisweet chocolate with extra sugar added. I have not used German chocolate in this book but, rather, have added extra reduced calorie sweeteners to baking chocolate or semisweet chocolate to give the same flavor as German chocolate.

Milk chocolate is a sweet chocolate with milk added and is the chocolate used in most candy bars.

Semisweet chocolate is baking chocolate with extra cocoa butter and flavorings. We commonly use chips or bits of this type of chocolate. Chocolate sprinkles, jimmies, shot or mounties are all considered chips or bits.

White chocolate, confectionary coating, dietetic white dipping or coating chocolate are imitation chocolates in which all or most of the cocoa butter has been replaced with another vegetable fat. It can be bought colored or can be colored and flavored at home with colored food oils.

Working with Chocolate

Melt chocolate slowly because it scorches easily. It is best melted over simmering water, never boiling water. You can use the top of a double boiler or a cup or bowl in a saucepan with a water bath. But keep your water only warm to prevent steam from getting into your chocolate. Chocolate can also be melted in your microwave, but you must do the melting process on low and check your chocolate often. Chocolate will harden again when cool and may be saved to use for another time.

Grate or chop chocolate easily when the chocolate is cool and firm.

Store chocolate in a cool, dry place. Chocolate is very sensitive to temperature changes. Allow chocolate to return to room temperature before heating or melting. If your chocolate develops a white film, do not despair; the film will leave as soon as the chocolate is melted.

Using the Recipes for Your Diet

All recipes have been developed using diet substitutions for sugar, syrup, sugared toppings, puddings and gelatins. Imitation or low-cal dairy and nondairy products are used in the recipes.

Read the recipes carefully, then assemble all equipment and ingredients. Use standard measuring equipment (whether metric or customary); be sure to measure accurately. Remember, these recipes are good for *everyone*, not just the diabetic. All liquids—milk, water, etc.—used in recipes are *cold* unless otherwise noted. All recipes found in this book are capitalized. Check the index for page numbers when specific recipes call for recipes, such as Semisweet Dipping Chocolate.

Customary Terms

t.	teaspoon
T.	tablespoon
c.	cup
env.	envelope
pkg.	package
pt.	pint
qt.	quart
oz.	ounce
lb.	pound
°F	degrees Fahrenheit
in.	inch

Metric Symbols

mL	millilitre
L	litre
g	gram
kg	kilogram
°C	degrees Celsius
mm	millimetre
cm	centimetre

Cooking Pans and Casseroles

CUSTOMARY	METRIC
1 qt.	1 L
2 qt.	2 L
3 qt.	3 L

Oven Cooking Guides

FAHRENHEIT °F	OVEN HEAT	CELSIUS °C
250–275°	Very slow	120–135°
300–325°	Slow	150–165°
350–375°	Moderate	175–190°
400–425°	Hot	200–220°
450–475°	Very hot	230–245°
475–500°	Hottest	250–290°

Candy Thermometer Guide

Use this guide to test for doneness:

FAHRENHEIT °F	TEST	CELSIUS °C
230–234°	Syrup: thread	100–112°
234–240°	Fondant/Fudge: soft ball	112–115°
244-248°	Caramels: firm ball	118–120°
250–266°	Marshmallows: hard ball	121–130°
270–290°	Taffy: soft crack	132–143°
300–310°	Brittle: hard crack	149–154°

Guide to Approximate Equivalents

	CUSTOMARY			METRIC	
Ounces Pounds	Cups	Tablespoons	Teaspoons	Millilitres	Grams Kilograms
			¼ t.	1 mL	1 g
			½ t.	2 mL	
			1 t.	5 mL	
			2 t.	10 mL	
½ oz.		1 T.	3 t.	15 mL	15 g
1 oz.		2 T.	6 t.	30 mL	30 g
2 oz.	¼ c.	4 T.	12 t.	60 mL	
4 oz.	½ c.	8 T.	24 t.	125 mL	
8 oz.	1 c.	16 T.	48 t.	250 mL	
2.2 lb.					1 kg
	4 c.			1 L	

Keep in mind that this is not an exact conversion, but, generally, may be used for food measurement. Also, some weights (ounces and grams) taken from manufacturers' packages may not be consistent or standard.

Guide to Pan Sizes

CUSTOMARY	HOLDS	METRIC	HOLDS
8-in. pie	2 c.	20-cm pie	600 mL
9-in. pie	1 qt.	23-cm pie	1 L
10-in. pie	1¼ qt.	25-cm pie	1.3 L
8-in. round	1 qt.	20-cm round	1 L
9-in. round	1½ qt.	23-cm round	1.5 L
8-in. square	2 qt.	20-cm square	2 L
9-in. square	2½ qt.	23-cm square	2.5 L
9 × 5 × 2-in. (loaf)	2 qt.	23 × 13 × 5-cm (loaf)	2 L
9-in. tube	3 qt.	23-cm tube	3 L
10-in. tube	3 qt.	25-cm tube	3 L
10-in. Bundt	3 qt.	25-cm Bundt	3 L
9 × 5 in.	1½ qt.	23 × 13 cm	1.5 L
10 × 6 in.	3½ qt.	25 × 16 cm	3.5 L
11 × 7 in.	3½ qt.	27 × 17 cm	3.5 L
13 × 9 × 2 in.	3½ qt.	33 × 23 × 5 cm	3.5 L
14 × 10 in.	cookie tin	36 × 25 cm	
15½ × 10½ × 1 in.	jelly roll	39 × 25 × 3 cm	

Candy, Fudge and More Candy

Basic Crème Center

3 oz.	cream cheese, softened	90 g
1 c.	Powdered Sugar Replacement	250 mL
2 T.	water	30 mL
1 t.	vanilla extract	5 mL

Beat cream cheese until fluffy. Stir in sugar replacement, water and vanilla extract. (Dough may be divided into parts and different flavorings and/or food color added to each part as suggested in various recipes.) Knead or work with the hand until dough is smooth. Use as directed in the recipes.

Yield: 1 c. (250 mL)
Exchange, full recipe: 4 fruit
6 fat
Calories, full recipe: 600

Powdered Sugar Replacement

2 c.	nonfat dry milk powder	500 mL
2 c.	cornstarch	500 mL
1 c.	granulated sugar replacement	250 mL

Combine all ingredients in food processor or blender. Whip until well blended and powdered.

Yield: 4 c. (1 L)
Exchange, ¼ c. (60 mL): 1 bread or ½ nonfat milk + ½ bread
Calories, ¼ c. (60 mL): 81

Semisweet Dipping Chocolate

1 c.	nonfat dry milk powder	250 mL
⅓ c.	cocoa	90 mL
2 T.	paraffin wax	30 mL
½ c.	water	125 mL
1 T.	vegetable oil	15 mL
1 T.	liquid sugar replacement	15 mL

Combine milk powder, cocoa and wax in food processor or blender; blend to the consistency of soft powder. Pour into top of double boiler and add water, stirring to blend. Add liquid shortening. Place over hot (not boiling) water, and cook and stir until wax pieces are completely dissolved and mixture thick, smooth and creamy. Remove from heat. Stir in sugar replacement and cool slightly. Dip candies according to recipe directions. Shake off excess chocolate. Place on very lightly greased waxed paper and allow to cool completely. (If candies do not remove easily, slightly warm the waxed paper over electric burner or with clothes iron.) Store in a cool place.

Yield: 1 c. (250 mL)
Exchange, full recipe: 3 low-fat milk
Calories, full recipe: 427

Quick No-Cook Fondant

Easy—and I like easy.

7 oz.	low-cal white frosting mix	200 g
2 T.	margarine	30 mL
1 to 2 T.	water	30 to 60 mL

Combine frosting mix and margarine in food processor or bowl. Work with steel blade or spoon until mixture is well blended. (Add very small amounts of water if needed.) Mixture will be very stiff at first; work and knead until mixture is well blended and smooth. Use as directed in recipe.

Yield: 1 c. (250 mL)
Exchange, full recipe: 7 bread
                           16 fat
Calories, full recipe: 1,200

Fast Holiday Drops

1 env.	unflavored gelatin	1 env.
⅔ c.	skim milk	180 mL
30	soda crackers, crumbed	30
½ c.	pecans, chopped fine	125 mL
1 t.	vanilla extract	5 mL
⅓ c.	creamy peanut butter	90 mL
⅓ c.	mini chocolate chips	90 mL

Soak gelatin in milk for 5 minutes; heat and stir until gelatin is dissolved and mixture boils. Remove from heat and quickly add remaining ingredients. Beat with a wooden spoon until mixture is thick enough to drop from a teaspoon onto waxed paper. Make 24 drops. Refrigerate until firm.

Yield: 24 drops
Exchange, 1 drop: ½ bread
1 fat
Calories, 1 drop: 76

Out-of-Bounds Candy Bars

Coconut and chocolate—a popular American combination.

1¼ c.	unsweetened coconut	310 mL
½ c.	milk	125 mL
2 t.	unflavored gelatin	10 mL
1 t.	cornstarch	5 mL
1 t.	white vanilla extract	5 mL
1 recipe	Semisweet Dipping Chocolate	1 recipe

Combine ¼ c. (60 mL) of the coconut, the milk, gelatin and cornstarch in blender; blend until smooth. Pour into small saucepan, cook and stir over medium heat until slightly thickened. Remove from heat and stir in vanilla and remaining coconut. Form into 8 bars, allow to firm and cool completely. Dip in chocolate.

Yield: 8 bars
Exchange, 1 bar: ⅔ full-fat milk
1 fat
Calories, 1 bar: 133

Butter Sticks

7 large	shredded wheat biscuits	7 large
½ c.	crunchy peanut butter	125 mL
3 T.	granulated sugar replacement	45 mL
2	egg whites	2
1 T.	flour	15 mL
1 T.	water	15 mL
1 t.	baking powder	5 mL
1 t.	vanilla extract	5 mL
1 recipe	Semisweet Dipping Chocolate	1 recipe

Break biscuits into large bowl or food processor. Add peanut butter, sugar replacement, egg whites, flour, water, baking powder and vanilla. Work with wooden spoon or steel blade until mixture is completely blended; mixture will be sticky. Form into 16 sticks and place them on an ungreased cookie sheet. Bake at 400 °F (200 °C) for 10 minutes, or until surface feels hard. Remove; cool slightly. Dip in chocolate.

Yield: 16 sticks
Exchange, 1 stick: ⅔ bread
Calories, 1 stick: 115

Rum Rounds

⅓ c.	Quick No-Cook Fondant	90 mL
1 t.	rum flavoring	5 mL
1 oz.	white dietetic chocolate coating	30 g

Work together fondant and rum flavoring until completely blended. Divide mixture in half. Form into two 5½ × ½-in. (14 × 1.3-cm) rolls. Cut into ¼-in. (6-mm) round discs. Place on plate and refrigerate until firm. Melt white dietetic chocolate coating in small custard cup over simmering water. Using two forks, dip rounds one at a time. Pick rounds out of the melted chocolate and place on waxed paper to dry. Refrigerate until very firm. Remove chocolate coating from heat; reserve. When rounds are firm, remelt any remaining chocolate and redip rounds.

Yield: 34 rounds
Exchange, 1 round: ⅓ fat
Calories, 1 round: 17

Chocolate Pudding Squares

A candy for pudding fans.

3 env.	unflavored gelatin	3 env.
1 c.	cold water	250 mL
2 T.	cocoa	30 mL
1 oz.	paraffin wax, grated	30 g
2 T.	flour	30 mL
1 c.	skim milk	250 mL
3 T.	margarine	45 mL

Combine unflavored gelatin and cold water in bowl; stir to mix. Set aside. Combine cocoa, wax, flour and skim milk in heavy saucepan; cook and stir until wax has melted and mixture is thick and smooth. Add softened gelatin. Cook and stir until mixture is thick. Remove from heat and add margarine. Stir to completely dissolve. Pour into lightly greased 9-in. (23-cm) square pan. Refrigerate until completely set. Cut into 1-in. (2.5-cm) squares. Refrigerate.

Yield: 81 pieces
Exchange, 1 piece: negligible
Calories, 1 piece: 3

Chocolate Butter Creams

1/4 c.	unsalted butter	60 mL
2 T.	skim milk	30 mL
1 t.	vanilla extract	5 mL
1 c.	Powdered Sugar Replacement	250 mL
1 recipe	Semisweet Dipping Chocolate	1 recipe

Beat together until fluffy the butter, milk and vanilla extract. Stir in sugar replacement. Knead or work with hands until smooth. Roll into small, marble-size balls; refrigerate until firm. Dip into melted dipping chocolate. Place on waxed paper to dry.

Yield: 45 creams
Exchange, 1 cream: ½ fat
Calories, 1 cream: 20

Date Surprise

You may tint white chocolate with small amount of food coloring.

50	dates, pitted	50
100	salted peanuts, whole	100
2 oz.	white dietetic chocolate coating	60 g
¼ oz.	paraffin wax	8 g

Remove any stem ends from dates. Carefully open each date and stuff with two whole peanuts. Place on a plate and refrigerate until cool. Melt white coating and paraffin wax in a small jar or dish over simmering water. Using two forks, dip each date, one at a time, until completely coated. Place on waxed paper to firm. Store in refrigerator.

Yield: 50 pieces
Exchange, 1 piece: ½ bread
Calories, 1 piece: 45

Fancy Prunes

Choose soft prunes for this candy.

48	dried prunes	48
24	walnut halves	24
¼ c.	Basic Crème Center	60 mL
½ recipe	Semisweet Dipping Chocolate	½ recipe

Slit sides of prunes and carefully remove the pits. Break walnut halves in half lengthwise. Wrap equal amounts of crème center around each section of walnut. Stuff a covered walnut into each prune cavity. Place on waxed paper on a plate. Refrigerate. Allow to chill at least 4 hours or overnight. When cold, dip in the chocolate. Place on waxed paper until firm. Store in refrigerator.

Yield: 48 pieces
Exchange, 1 piece: ½ bread
Calories, 1 piece: 35

Triple C Treat

40	Bing cherries	40
1 c.	unsweetened coconut, grated	250 mL
½ c.	skim milk	125 mL
2 t.	unflavored gelatin	10 mL
2 t.	cornstarch	10 mL
2 t.	coconut flavoring	10 mL
1 oz.	dietetic chocolate coating	30 g
1 oz.	white dietetic dipping chocolate	30 g

Carefully pit the cherries. Set in refrigerator to chill. Combine unsweetened coconut, skim milk, gelatin, cornstarch and coconut flavoring in saucepan and stir to blend. Set aside for 5 minutes to allow gelatin to soften. Cook and stir over low heat until mixture is very thick. Remove from heat and allow to cool. Divide in half. Form 40 pea-size balls of the coconut mixture and push one ball into each cherry center. Cover cherries with remaining coconut mixture. Place on plate and refrigerate to firm. Melt chocolate coating in small custard cup and dip one-half of each cherry. Place on waxed paper to harden. Melt white chocolate in another custard cup and dip the other side of each cherry. Place on waxed paper to harden. Store in refrigerator.

Yield: 40 pieces
Exchange, 1 piece: ⅕ bread
Calories, 1 piece: 20

Chocolate-Coated Cherries

A quick candy.

1 recipe	Basic Crème Center	1 recipe
30	Bing cherries, including pits and stems	30
½ recipe	Semisweet Dipping Chocolate	½ recipe

Wrap Basic Crème Center dough around each cherry; chill thoroughly. Dip in chocolate and dry completely.

Yield: 30 cherries
Exchange, 1 cherry: ⅕ bread
½ fat
Calories, 1 cherry: 31

Apricot Nuggets

Elegant candy to delight your guests.

1 env.	unflavored gelatin	1 env.
¼ c.	water	60 mL
1½ c.	dried apricots	375 mL
1 T.	flour	15 mL
2 T.	orange peel, grated	30 mL
1 t.	vanilla extract	5 mL
2 oz.	dietetic chocolate coating, melted	60 g

Sprinkle gelatin over water; allow to soften for 5 minutes. Heat and stir until gelatin is completely dissolved. Combine apricots, flour, orange peel in blender or food processor and work until finely chopped. Add apricot mixture to gelatin. Add vanilla extract and stir to completely blend. Line with plastic wrap or waxed paper an 8-in. (20-cm) square pan. Spread fruit mixture evenly into pan and set aside until cool and completely firm. Turn out onto a cutting board. Cut into 1-in. (2.5-cm) squares. Place on plate in refrigerator until chilled. Dip in melted dietetic chocolate.

Yield: 64 nuggets
Exchange, 1 nugget: ⅓ bread
Calories, 1 nugget: 14

Sweet Chocolate-Covered Pineapple

⅓ c.	Quick No-Cook Fondant	90 mL
18	bite-size pineapple tidbits in their own juice	18
1 oz.	dietetic chocolate coating	30 g

Drain pineapple tidbits thoroughly. Place on paper towel, drain for 10 to 15 minutes and pat until slightly dry. Form 1 t. (5 mL) of fondant mixture around each pineapple tidbit. Place on plate and refrigerate until firm. Melt chocolate coating in a small custard cup over simmering water. Using two forks, dip each pineapple bit, one at a time, in the chocolate. Remove and place on waxed paper and allow to harden. Store in refrigerator.

Yield: 18 pieces
Exchange, 1 piece: ⅓ fruit
½ fat
Calories, 1 piece: 32

Raisin Balls

1 env.	unflavored gelatin	1 env.
¼ c.	apple juice	60 mL
2 c.	raisins	500 mL
2 T.	flour	30 mL
½ c.	walnuts, finely chopped	125 mL
½ c.	semisweet chocolate chips	125 mL
¼ oz.	paraffin wax	8 g

Sprinkle gelatin over apple juice; allow to soften for 5 minutes. Heat and stir until gelatin is completely dissolved. Combine raisins and flour in a mixing bowl; toss to completely coat. Stir in walnuts. Add raisin mixture to apple-gelatin. Stir to thoroughly blend. Remove from heat and allow to cool. Form into 30 balls. Refrigerate until firm. Melt chocolate chips and wax in small pan or bowl over simmering water. Dip chilled raisin balls in chocolate. Place on waxed paper until firm. Store in refrigerator.

Yield: 30 balls
Exchange, 1 ball: ½ bread
½ fat
Calories, 1 ball: 56

Mint Mounds

⅓ c.	Quick No-Cook Fondant	90 mL
½ t.	wintergreen flavoring	2 mL
2 drops	green food coloring	2 drops
1 oz.	dietetic chocolate coating	30 g
¼ oz.	paraffin wax	8 g

Combine fondant, flavoring and food coloring; mix until color is completely blended in fondant. Cover a ½ t. (2 mL) spoon with plastic wrap, press a small amount of fondant mixture into plastic on spoon to make a mound. Remove and place on plate. Repeat with remaining fondant. Refrigerate until Firm. Melt dietetic chocolate coating and wax in a small custard cup over simmering water. Remove and discard plastic wrap from mounds. Using two forks, dip mounds one at a time. Pick mounds out of melted chocolate and place on waxed paper to dry.

Yield: 26
Exchange, 1 mound: ½ fat
Calories, 1 mound: 22

Double-Fudge Balls

⅓ c.	margarine, softened	90 mL
3 T.	skim evaporated milk	45 mL
dash	salt	dash
1 t.	vanilla extract	5 mL
¼ c.	cocoa	60 mL
1 c.	Powdered Sugar Replacement	250 mL
1 recipe	Semisweet Dipping Chocolate	1 recipe

Cream together until fluffy the margarine, milk, salt and vanilla. Stir in cocoa and sugar replacement. Knead until dough is smooth; shape dough into 60 small balls. Dip balls in chocolate; cool completely, then dip again and cool.

Yield: 60 balls
Exchange, 1 ball: ⅓ bread
½ fat
Calories, 1 ball: 50

Fudge Candy

13-oz. can	skim evaporated milk	385-mL can
3 T.	cocoa	45 mL
¼ c.	butter	60 mL
1 T.	granulated sugar replacement	15 mL
dash	salt	dash
1 t.	vanilla extract	5 mL
2½ c.	unsweetened cereal crumbs	625 mL
¼ c.	nuts, very finely chopped	60 mL

Combine milk and cocoa in saucepan; cook and beat over low heat until cocoa is dissolved. Add butter, sugar replacement, salt and vanilla. Bring to a boil; reduce heat and cook for 2 minutes. Remove from heat; add cereal crumbs and work in with wooden spoon. Cool 15 minutes. Divide in half; roll each half into a tube, 8 in. (20 cm) long. Roll each tube in finely chopped nuts. Wrap in waxed paper; chill overnight. Cut into ¼-in. (6-mm) slices.

Yield: 64 slices
Exchange, 2 slices: ½ bread
½ fat
Calories, 2 slices: 60

Butterscotch-Chocolate Fudge

13-oz. can	skim evaporated milk	385-g can
1 c.	water	250 mL
¼ c.	cornstarch	60 mL
3 T.	granulated sugar replacement	45 mL
½ c.	chocolate chips	125 mL
½ c.	butterscotch chips	125 mL
1 t.	vanilla extract	5 mL
½ c.	walnuts, chopped	125 mL

Combine evaporated milk, water, cornstarch, sugar replacement, chocolate chips and butterscotch chips in saucepan. Cook and stir over medium heat until mixture thickens and chips are melted. Cool. Stir in vanilla extract. Beat with an electric mixer until light. Stir in walnuts. Turn into buttered 9-in. (23-cm) square baking dish. Spread evenly. Cool and cut in 1-in. (2.5-cm) squares.

Yield: 81
Exchange, 1 square: ⅕ bread
⅕ fat
Calories, 1 square: 21

French Fudge

Do you like fudge extra rich?

13 oz. can	skim evaporated milk	385-g can
2 T.	cornstarch	30 mL
1 T.	liquid sugar replacement	15 mL
½ c.	chocolate chips	125 mL
3 oz.	cream cheese, softened	90 g
1½ t.	vanilla extract	7 mL

Combine evaporated milk, cornstarch, sugar replacement and chocolate chips in saucepan. Cook and stir until mixture is thick and chocolate chips are melted. Whip cream cheese until light and fluffy. Beat in chocolate/milk mixture. Stir in vanilla extract. Turn into buttered 8-in. (20-cm) square baking dish. Chill until firm. Cut into 1-in. (2.5-cm) squares. Store in refrigerator.

Yield: 64 pieces
Exchange, 1 piece: ¼ bread
Calories, 1 piece: 18

Maple-Pecan Centers

1/3 c.	Quick No-Cook Fondant	90 mL
1/2 t.	maple flavoring	2 mL
1/4 c.	pecans, finely chopped	60 mL
1 oz.	dietetic chocolate coating	30 g

Combine fondant and maple flavoring in bowl and mix until completely blended. Work in the pecans. Set aside until mixture is slightly firm. Form into 20 small balls. Place on plate in refrigerator until firm. Melt chocolate coating in small custard cup over simmering water. Dip each ball in chocolate; set on waxed paper to harden.

Yield: 20 pieces
Exchange, 1 piece: 1/5 bread
1/2 fat
Calories, 1 piece: 38

Mock Turtles

18	pecan halves	18
1/2 c.	cold water	125 mL
1 env.	unflavored gelatin	1 env.
1/2 c.	skim milk	125 mL
1 T.	granulated sugar replacement	15 mL
1/2 t.	maple flavoring	2 mL
1 oz.	dietetic chocolate coating	30 g

Place a pecan half in bottom on petit four cup. Place petit four cup into small nut cup or mini muffin tin. (This is to keep the petit four cup in shape.) Combine cold water and gelatin in saucepan; allow to rest for 5 minutes. Cook and stir over medium heat until mixture comes to full boil; boil for 2 minutes. Remove from heat. Stir in milk, sugar replacement and maple flavoring to thoroughly blend. Set aside until mixture is the consistency of thick syrup. Spoon 2 t. (10 mL) of maple mixture over pecan in petit four cup. Chill until firm. Melt chocolate coating in small custard cup over simmering water. Divide melted chocolate evenly among the 18 petit four cups. Store in refrigerator.

Yield: 18
Exchange, 1 turtle: 1/5 bread
Calories, 1 turtle: 16

Almond Squares

9	graham crackers	9
1/3 c.	almonds, slivered and toasted	90 mL
1/2 c.	unsalted butter	125 mL
3 T.	granulated brown sugar replacement	45 mL
1/4 t.	almond flavoring	1 mL
1/3 c.	chocolate chips	90 mL

Arrange graham crackers on bottom of greased 9-in. (23-cm) baking dish. Sprinkle with almonds. Melt butter in small frying pan. Cook until butter is slightly brown, add brown sugar replacement and stir to mix. Remove from heat and add almond flavoring. Pour over graham crackers. Bake at 325 °F (165 °C) for 10 minutes. Remove from oven. Sprinkle with chocolate chips. Allow to cool 10 to 12 minutes and cut into 1-in. (2.5-cm) squares.

Yield: 81 squares
Exchange, 1 square: 2/5 fat
Calories, 1 square: 19

Peanut Favorites

1 env.	unflavored gelatin	1 env.
1/4 c.	skim milk	60 mL
1/2 c.	chunky peanut butter	125 mL
3/4 c.	unsalted peanuts, chopped	190 mL
1/2 c.	no-sugar wheat flakes	125 mL
2 oz.	dietetic chocolate coating	60 g
1/4 oz.	paraffin wax	8 g

Soak gelatin in cold milk in saucepan, allow to soften for 5 minutes. Add peanut butter. Cook and stir over medium heat until peanut butter is melted and mixture is very hot. Remove from heat and allow to cool slightly. Stir in peanuts and wheat flakes. Form into 28 finger-like shapes. Place on a plate and refrigerate until cool and set. Melt chocolate coating and wax in small pan or bowl over simmering water. Dip peanut fingers, one at a time. Place on waxed paper to cool.

Yield: 28 fingers
Exchange, 1 finger: 1/4 bread
1 fat
Calories, 1 finger: 63

Marble Creams

9	graham crackers	9
1 c.	cold water	250 mL
2 pkg.	unflavored gelatin	2 pkg.
2 T.	flour	30 mL
2 T.	cornstarch	30 mL
½ t.	cream of tartar	2 mL
⅓ c.	dietetic maple syrup	90 mL
¼ t.	baking soda	1 mL
⅓ c.	chocolate chips	90 mL

Arrange graham crackers in the bottom of a greased 9-in. (23-cm) square baking dish. Set aside. Combine cold water and gelatin in a saucepan; allow to soften for 5 minutes. Stir in flour, cornstarch, cream of tartar and maple syrup. Cook and stir over medium heat until mixture is very thick. Remove from heat and beat in baking soda. Cool slightly, pour mixture over graham crackers. Sprinkle with chocolate chips. With the tip of a knife, carefully swirl melting chips into maple mixture. Refrigerate until firm. With a sharp knife, cut into 1-in. (2.5-cm) squares.

Yield: 81 squares
Exchange, 2 squares: ⅕ bread
Calories, 2 squares: 17

Chocolate Crunch Candy

1 c.	nonfat dry milk powder	250 mL
½ c.	cocoa	125 mL
2 T.	liquid fructose	30 mL
3 T.	water	45 mL
1½ c.	chow mein noodles	375 mL

Combine milk powder and cocoa in food processor or blender; blend to a fine powder. Stir in fructose and water and beat until smooth and creamy. Slightly crush the chow mein noodles and fold them into chocolate mixture. Drop by teaspoonfuls onto waxed paper. Cool at room temperature.

Yield: 30 pieces
Exchange, 1 piece: ⅓ bread
Calories, 1 piece: 11

Walnut Riches

1 recipe	Basic Crème Center	1 recipe
2 t.	brandy flavoring	10 mL
¼ c.	mini chocolate chips	60 mL
2 oz.	dietetic chocolate coating	60 g
¼ oz.	paraffin wax	8 g
35	walnut halves, roasted	35

Combine crème center dough and brandy flavoring in a mixing bowl. Work with your hands until mixture is well blended. Work in chocolate chips. Divide mixture into 70 small pieces and form into desired shapes. Place on plate and refrigerate until firm. Melt chocolate coating and wax in a small custard cup over simmering water. Using two forks, dip each shape one at a time in the chocolate. Remove and place on waxed paper. Break each walnut in half lengthwise and place each of these walnut quarters lengthwise on each candy. Cool.

Yield: 70 pieces
Exchange, 1 piece: ½ fat
Calories, 1 piece: 22

Candy and Then Some

1 env.	unflavored gelatin	1 env.
¼ c.	water	60 mL
½ c.	dried apricots	125 mL
½ c.	dates, chopped	125 mL
½ c.	white raisins	125 mL
½ c.	dried apples	125 mL
¼ c.	pecans	60 mL
¼ c.	walnuts	60 mL
2 T.	flour	30 mL
2 t.	brandy flavoring	10 mL
1 recipe	Semisweet Dipping Chocolate	1 recipe

Soak gelatin in water for 5 minutes; heat and stir until gelatin is dissolved. Combine remaining ingredients in food processor and work with an on/off method until fruits are finely chopped. Stir into gelatin mixture until completely coated. Form into 40 balls. Place on plate and refrigerate until firm. Dip in semisweet dipping chocolate.

Yield: 40 balls
Exchange, 1 ball: 1 fruit
Calories, 1 ball: 40

Plain and Fancy Cookies

Peanut Whirlwinds

Attractive and easy.

½ c.	butter, softened	125 mL
⅓ c.	shortening, softened	90 mL
3 oz.	cream cheese, softened	85 g
½ c.	granulated sugar replacement	125 mL
2 t.	vanilla extract	10 mL
2 c.	all-purpose flour, sifted	500 mL
½ t.	salt	2 mL
½ c.	chocolate chips, melted	125 mL
2 T.	butter, melted	30 mL
⅓ c.	unsalted peanuts, finely ground	90 mL

Combine butter, shortening, cream cheese, sugar replacement and vanilla extract in mixing bowl. Beat until smooth and creamy. Stir in flour and salt until completely blended. Refrigerate at least 2 hours until easy to handle. On lightly floured surface, roll half of dough to ⅛-in. (3-mm) thickness. Mix together melted chocolate chips, butter and ground peanuts to make a paste. Spread half of the chocolate paste over rolled dough. Roll up, jelly-roll style. Repeat with remaining dough. With a sharp knife, cut into ⅛-in. (3-mm) slices. Place on greased cookie sheets, 1 in. (2.5 cm) apart. Bake at 400 °F (200 °C) for 8 to 10 minutes.

Yield: 96 cookies
Exchange, 1 cookie: ¼ bread
⅓ fat
Calories, 1 cookie: 29

Chocolate Sandies

¾ c.	butter, softened	190 mL
1 oz.	baking chocolate, melted	30 g
¼ c.	granulated sugar replacement	60 mL
1 T.	water	15 mL
1 T.	vanilla extract	15 mL
2 c.	flour, sifted	500 mL
½ c.	pecans, finely ground	125 mL

Cream butter, melted chocolate and sugar replacement; add water and vanilla extract and mix well. Blend in flour and pecans. Chill at least 4 hours or overnight. Shape into balls. Bake on ungreased cookie sheet at 325 °F (165 °C) for 15 to 20 minutes. Remove from pan immediately.

Yield: 40 cookies
Exchange, 1 cookie: ⅓ bread
                        1 fat
Calories, 1 cookie: 66

Applesauce Cocoa Cookies

½ c.	vegetable shortening, softened	125 mL
⅓ c.	granulated sugar replacement	90 mL
1	egg, beaten	1
2 c.	cake flour	500 mL
⅓ c.	cocoa	90 mL
½ t.	cinnamon	2 mL
½ t.	salt	2 mL
½ t.	baking soda	2 mL
1 t.	baking powder	5 mL
1 c.	unsweetened applesauce	250 mL
¼ c.	water	60 mL

Cream together the shortening and sugar replacement. Add egg and blend well. Sift all dry ingredients together and add alternately with applesauce and water to creamed mixture. Be sure to add flour first and last. Drop by teaspoon onto greased cookie sheet. Bake at 375 °F (190 °C) for 12 to 15 minutes.

Yield: 40 cookies
Exchange, 1 cookie: ⅓ bread
                        ⅗ fat
Calories, 1 cookie: 47

Chocolate Rosettes

2	eggs	2
1 c.	skim milk	250 mL
¾ c.	flour	190 mL
¼ c.	cocoa	60 mL
2 T.	sorbitol	30 mL
dash	salt	dash
	Powdered Sugar Replacement	

In a blender or mixing bowl, beat eggs and milk together until frothy. Add flour, cocoa, sorbitol and salt. Beat until smooth. Chill for one hour.

Dip and heat a rosette iron in deep fat heated to 375 °F (175 °C). Remove iron and drain slightly on absorbent paper. Dip iron into batter only to depth of the form—not over the top. (Excess batter will have to be removed after frying, before the rosettes can be taken off the form.) Lower iron into the fat and fry the rosette until golden brown. Drain on absorbent paper. Remove rosette from the iron. Continue until all rosettes have been fried. Store in tight container in dry place or freeze. Sprinkle with powdered sugar replacement before serving.

Yield: 30 rosettes
Exchange, 1 rosette: ⅔ bread
                      ⅓ fat
Calories, 1 rosette: 40

Fun Form Cookies

All kids like form cookies and chocolate makes them better.

⅓ c.	margarine, softened	90 mL
½ c.	liquid fructose	125 mL
1	egg, slightly beaten	1
1 t.	rum flavoring	5 mL
2 c.	all-purpose flour	500 mL
2 t.	baking powder	10 mL
¼ t.	salt	1 mL
1 oz.	baking chocolate, melted	30 g

Combine margarine and fructose in mixing bowl, beat until smooth and creamy. Add egg and rum flavoring and beat well. Sift flour, baking powder and salt together. Stir into creamed mixture. Divide dough in half. To one half of dough, work in the melted chocolate. Combine white and chocolate doughs and work with your hands to **slightly** mix doughs. Wrap in plastic wrap and refrigerate overnight. Roll out to ⅛-in. (3-mm) thickness. Cut into 2-in. (5-cm) decorative shapes. Place on ungreased cookie sheets. Bake at 400 °F (200 °C) for 8 to 10 minutes.

Yield: 72 cookies
Exchange, 1 cookie: ⅓ bread
⅓ fat
Calories, 1 cookie: 26

Chocolate Chewies

A chocolate-covered raisin cookie.

1½ oz.	baking chocolate	45 mL
½ c.	butter	125 mL
2 T.	boiling water	30 mL
¼ c.	chopped raisins	60 mL
3	eggs	3
⅓ c.	granulated sugar replacement	90 mL
¾ c.	flour	190 mL
½ t.	baking powder	2 mL
½ t.	salt	2 mL
dash	nutmeg	dash

Melt chocolate and butter in top of double boiler over simmering water. In a small bowl, pour boiling water over raisins. Set aside and stir occasionally to plump the raisins. Beat eggs and sugar replacement until light and fluffy; add chocolate mixture. Sift together the flour, baking powder, salt and nutmeg. Blend into creamed mixture. Fold in plumped raisins with water. Chill at least 2 hours. Drop by teaspoonfuls onto greased cookie sheets. Bake at 350 °F (175 °C) for 10 to 12 minutes.

Yield: 24 cookies
Exchange, 1 cookie: ⅓ bread
1 fat
Calories, 1 cookie: 72

Cornflake Macaroons

A favorite at bake sales.

2	egg whites	2
½ c.	granulated sugar replacement	125 mL
3 T.	sorbitol	45 mL
2 c.	cornflakes, unsweetened	500 mL
⅓ c.	mini chocolate chips	90 mL
½ c.	grated coconut, unsweetened	125 mL
½ t.	vanilla extract	2 mL

Beat egg whites until they are stiff enough to hold their shape but not until they lose their shiny appearance. Carefully, fold in remaining ingredients. Drop by teaspoonfuls onto a well-greased cookie sheet. Bake at 350 °F (175 °C) for 10 to 15 minutes or until done. Remove macaroons immediately with a spatula.

Yield: 24 cookies
Exchange, 1 cookie: ⅓ bread
⅓ fat
Calories, 1 cookie: 27

Cocoa Drops

1 c.	vegetable shortening, softened	250 mL
½ c.	granulated brown sugar replacement	125 mL
2	eggs	2
1¼ c.	skim milk	310 mL
2½ t.	vanilla extract	12 mL
4 c.	cake flour	1 L
1 t.	salt	5 mL
3 t.	baking powder	15 mL
¾ c.	cocoa	190 mL

Mix shortening and brown sugar replacement together. Add eggs and beat well. Combine milk and vanilla extract. Sift dry ingredients together and add alternately with milk to the batter. Drop by teaspoonfuls onto a greased cookie sheet. Bake at 350 °F (175 °C) for 10 to 12 minutes.

Yield: 120 cookies
Exchange, 1 cookie: ⅓ bread
⅓ fat
Calories, 1 cookie: 30

Chocolate Tea Cookies

¼ c.	vegetable shortening, soft	60 mL
3 T.	granulated sugar replacement	45 mL
1	egg	1
½ t.	vanilla extract	2 mL
2 T.	skim milk	30 mL
1¼ c.	cake flour, sifted	310 mL
1 oz.	baking chocolate, melted	30 g

Cream shortening. Add sugar replacement, egg, vanilla extract and milk. Blend well. Add half the sifted flour; stir to completely blend. Stir in melted chocolate and remaining flour. With cookie press, press onto ungreased cookie sheets. Bake at 350 °F (175 °C) for 20 minutes.

Yield: 36 cookies
Exchange, 1 cookie: ⅓ bread
⅓ fat
Calories, 1 cookie: 32

Rich Teas

A cookie to serve at parties.

½ c.	vegetable shortening, softened	125 mL
¼ c.	granulated sugar replacement	60 mL
1	egg, beaten	1
1 t.	vanilla extract	5 mL
½ t.	salt	2 mL
5 T.	skim milk	75 mL
2 c.	cake flour, sifted	500 mL
1½ oz.	baking chocolate	45 g

Cream shortening and sugar replacement. Add beaten egg, vanilla extract, salt and milk. Blend thoroughly and add half of the sifted flour. When well mixed, add melted chocolate and remaining flour. Mould with cookie press on cold, ungreased cookie sheet. Bake at 350 °F (175 °C) for 12 to 15 minutes.

Yield: 72 cookies
Exchange, 1 cookie: ¼ bread
⅓ fat
Calories, 1 cookie: 27

Chocolate Wafers

¼ c.	margarine, softened	60 mL
4 t.	granulated sugar replacement	20 mL
1	egg	1
2 T.	cocoa	30 mL
1 t.	vanilla extract	5 mL
1 c.	flour	250 mL
1 t.	baking powder	5 mL
¼ t.	baking soda	1 mL
dash	salt	dash
2 T.	water	30 mL

Combine margarine, sugar replacement, egg, cocoa and vanilla extract in mixing bowl or food processor. With electric mixer or steel blade, whip until creamy. Add flour, baking powder, baking soda, salt and water; mix well. Shape into 30 balls. Wrap in waxed paper or plastic wrap. Chill at least 1 hour or overnight. Remove wrap. Roll out dough to ⅛-in. (3-mm) thickness into round wafers, using a cookie cutter. Place on ungreased cookie sheets. Bake at 350 °F (175 °C) for 8 to 10 minutes.

Yield: 30 wafers
Exchange, 1 wafer: ⅓ vegetable
Calories, 1 wafer: 29

Pinwheels

½ c.	margarine, softened	125 mL
½ c.	granulated sugar replacement	125 mL
1 T.	vanilla extract	15 mL
1 T.	water	15 mL
1	egg	1
1⅔ c.	flour, sifted	410 mL
½ t.	baking powder	2 mL
½ t.	baking soda	2 mL
½	salt	2 mL
1 oz.	baking chocolate, melted	30 g

Cream margarine, sugar replacement, and vanilla extract until light and fluffy. Beat in water and egg. Sift together dry ingredients; blend into creamed mixture. Divide dough in half. Blend 1-oz. (30-g) of melted baking chocolate into one-half of dough. Thoroughly chill both dough halves. Roll each half of dough into a 10-in. (25-cm) square. Brush one layer with water, place other layer on top; roll up as for jelly roll. Cut into ⅛-in. (3-mm) slices. Bake at 375 °F (174 °C) for 6 to 8 minutes.

Yield: 80 cookies
Exchange, 2 cookies: ⅓ bread
⅗ fat
Calories, 2 cookies: 44

Peanut Butter Drops

1 c.	chunky peanut butter	250 mL
½ c.	butter	125 mL
1½ oz.	baking chocolate, melted	45 g
1 T.	vanilla extract	15 mL
3 T.	granulated sugar replacement	45 mL
2 T.	sorbitol	30 mL
¼ c.	liquid fructose	60 mL
2	eggs	2
2 T.	water	30 mL
2½ c.	flour	625 mL
1 t.	baking soda	5 mL

Cream together the peanut butter, butter, baking chocolate and vanilla extract. Gradually add sugar replacement, sorbitol and fructose. Continue beating and add eggs, one at a time, and beat well after each addition. Beat until light and fluffy. Sift together flour and baking soda. Add to creamed mixture and mix together thoroughly. Drop by teaspoonfuls onto ungreased cookie sheet. Bake at 375 °F (190 °C) for 10 to 12 minutes.

Yield: 96 cookies
Exchange, 1 cookie: ⅓ bread
½ fat
Calories, 1 cookie: 40

Chocolate Mounties

1 c.	vegetable shortening, softened	250 mL
1/2 c.	granulated brown sugar replacement	125 mL
2	eggs, well beaten	2
1 T.	vanilla extract	15 mL
3 T.	water	45 mL
3 1/2 c.	flour	875 mL
1 t.	salt	5 mL
2 t.	baking powder	10 mL
1 c.	skim milk	250 mL
3 oz.	baking chocolate, melted	90 g
1 c.	walnuts, coarsely chopped	250 mL

Cream shortening and sugar together. Add eggs, vanilla extract and water. Sift flour, salt and baking powder together and add alternately with the milk to the creamed mixture. Add melted chocolate and walnuts. Drop from a teaspoon onto a greased cookie sheet. Bake at 350 °F (175 °C) for 8 to 10 minutes.

Yield: 130 cookies
Exchange, 1 cookie: 1/5 bread
                          3/5 fat
Calories, 1 cookie: 36

Mocha Drops

1/2 c.	vegetable shortening	125 mL
1 1/2 oz.	baking chocolate	45 g
1/3 c.	brown sugar replacement	90 mL
1	egg	1
2 t.	vanilla extract	10 mL
1/2 c.	buttermilk	125 mL
3 T.	strong coffee	45 mL
1 1/3 c.	flour	340 mL
1/2 t.	baking powder	2 mL
1/2 t.	baking soda	2 mL
1/4 t.	salt	1 mL
1/4 c.	walnuts, chopped	60 mL

Melt shortening and baking chocolate together in a saucepan. Cool 5 minutes. Stir in brown sugar replacement. Beat in the egg, vanilla extract, buttermilk and coffee. Sift together dry ingredients and add to chocolate mixture. Stir in walnuts. Drop from teaspoon onto greased cookie sheet. Bake at 375 °F (190 °C) for 8 to 10 minutes.

Yield: 50 cookies
Exchange, 1 cookie: ⅕ bread
⅗ fat
Calories, 1 cookie: 40

Fructose-Chocolate-Oatmeal Cookies

Freeze batches of these for Christmas.

2½ c.	*cake flour*	*625 mL*
1 t.	*baking powder*	*5 mL*
¼ t.	*baking soda*	*1 mL*
½ t.	*salt*	*2 mL*
1 t.	*cinnamon*	*5 mL*
1 c.	*vegetable shortening, softened*	*250 mL*
½ c.	*liquid fructose*	*125 mL*
2	*eggs, beaten*	*2*
2 oz.	*baking chocolate, melted*	*60 g*
1½ c.	*oatmeal*	*375 mL*

Sift cake flour, baking powder, baking soda, salt and cinnamon together. Cream shortening and fructose. Add beaten eggs, melted chocolate and oatmeal. Mix thoroughly. Add sifted dry ingredients. Drop from a teaspoon onto a greased cookie sheet. Bake at 325 °F (165 °C) for 15 to 20 minutes.

Yield: 66 cookies
Exchange, 1 cookie: ⅓ bread
⅗ fat
Calories, 1 cookie: 53

Banana Cookies

2¼ c.	flour	560 mL
2 t.	baking powder	10 mL
½ t.	salt	2 mL
¼ t.	baking soda	1 mL
⅓ c.	vegetable shortening, softened	90 mL
⅓ c.	granulated sugar replacement	90 mL
⅓ c.	cocoa	90 mL
2	eggs, beaten	2
½ t.	vanilla extract	2 mL
4	bananas, mashed	4

Sift dry ingredients together. Cream shortening, sugar replacement and cocoa thoroughly; add eggs and vanilla extract. Beat well. Add mashed bananas alternately with dry ingredients. Drop by teaspoonfuls onto greased cookie sheet. Bake at 350 °F (175 °C) for 12 to 15 minutes.

Yield: 60 cookies
Exchange, 1 cookie: ⅓ bread
⅖ fat
Calories, 1 cookie: 36

Walnut Wheels

A different chocolate walnut cookie.

⅓ c.	butter, softened	90 mL
½ c.	granulated sugar replacement	125 mL
1	egg	1
1 oz.	baking chocolate, melted	30 g
1 T.	warm water	15 mL
1 t.	vanilla extract	5 mL
⅔ c.	cake flour, sifted	180 mL
½ t.	baking powder	2 mL
¼ t.	salt	1 mL
24	walnut halves	24

Cream butter until light and fluffy, then beat in sugar replacement. Beat in egg, chocolate, warm water and vanilla extract. Stir in cake flour, baking powder and salt. Drop by teaspoonfuls onto greased baking sheet. Garnish each cookie with a walnut half. Bake at 350 °F (175 °C) for 8 to 10 minutes.

Yield: 24 cookies
Exchange, 1 cookie: ⅓ bread
                    ⅗ fat
Calories, 1 cookie: 40

Khip Kisses

Since I use block chocolate instead of chips, I call these "Khip Kisses."

2	egg whites	2
dash	salt	dash
⅛ t.	cream of tartar	½ mL
3 T.	granulated sugar replacement	45 mL
2 oz.	semisweet chocolate	60 g
¼ c.	walnuts, finely chopped	60 mL
1 t.	vanilla extract	5 mL

Beat egg whites until foamy, then add salt and cream of tartar. Continue beating until eggs are stiff but not dry. Add sugar replacement, beating thoroughly. Cut or grate chocolate into very small pieces. Fold in chocolate, walnuts and vanilla extract. Drop from a teaspoon onto ungreased heavy paper. Bake at 300 °F (150 °C) for 20 to 25 minutes. Remove from paper while slightly warm.

Yield: 18 kisses
Exchange, 1 kiss: ⅖ fat
Calories, 1 kiss: 28

German Crinkles

2 c.	flour	500 mL
2 t.	baking powder	10 mL
½ t.	salt	2 mL
½ c.	vegetable shortening, softened	125 mL
⅔ c.	granulated sugar replacement	160 mL
2 t.	vanilla extract	10 mL
2	eggs, slightly beaten	2
1½ oz.	baking chocolate, melted	45 mL
⅓ c.	skim milk	90 mL
1¼ c.	hazelnuts, finely ground	60 mL

Sift together flour, baking powder and salt. Set aside. Cream shortening, sugar replacement and vanilla extract. Beat in eggs and melted chocolate. Alternately, add flour mixture with milk to creamed mixture. Blend in hazelnuts. Chill 4 hours. Form into balls. Place on greased cookie sheet with space for cookies to spread. Bake at 350 °F (175 °C) for 12 to 15 minutes. Cool slightly; remove from pan.

Yield: 50 cookies
Exchange, 1 cookie: ¼ bread
                    ½ fat
Calories, 1 cookie: 47

Scottish Melts

3	eggs, beaten	3
½ c.	granulated sugar replacement	125 mL
¼ t.	salt	1 mL
3 T.	shortening, melted	45 mL
1 oz.	baking chocolate, melted	30 g
1 T.	vanilla extract	15 mL
3 c.	oatmeal	750 mL

Beat eggs, add sugar replacement gradually and beat well with each addition. Add salt, shortening, chocolate, vanilla extract and the oatmeal. Drop by teaspoonfuls onto greased cookie sheet. Bake at 325 °F (165 °C) for 17 to 25 minutes. Remove from pan while still warm.

Yield: 106 cookies
Exchange, 4 cookies: ⅕ bread
                      ½ fat
Calories, 4 cookies: 40

Quick Cookies

Citrus Cookies

8-oz. box	no-sugar chocolate cake mix	226-g box
4 t.	lemon peel, freshly grated	20 mL
2 t.	orange peel, freshly grated	10 mL
3 T.	orange juice	45 mL
1	egg white	1

Combine all ingredients in mixing bowl and beat at medium speed until mixture is smooth. Drop by teaspoonfuls onto greased cookie sheet. Bake at 350 °F (175 °C) for 8 to 10 minutes. Remove from pan immediately.

Yield: 60 cookies
Exchange, 1 cookie: ⅓ bread
Calories, 1 cookie: 15

Filbert Balls

8-oz. box	no-sugar chocolate cake mix	226-g box
1	egg yolk	1
2 t.	vanilla extract	10 mL
1	egg white	1
1 t.	water	5 mL
½ c.	filberts, finely ground	125 mL

Combine cake mix, egg yolk, water and vanilla extract in mixing bowl; beat until smooth. Refrigerate until easy to handle. Form dough by teaspoon into balls. Dip balls in mixture of beaten egg white and water; shake off excess. Then roll in ground filberts. Place on greased cookie sheet. Bake at 350 °F (175 °C) for 10 to 12 minutes.

Yield: 60 cookies
Exchange, 1 cookie: ⅓ bread
⅓ fat
Calories, 1 cookie: 22

Peanut Butter Drops

8-oz. box	no-sugar chocolate cake mix	226-g box
1/3 c.	peanut butter	90 mL
1	egg	1
4 t.	water	20 mL
1 T.	margarine, softened	15 mL

Combine one-half of cake mix, peanut butter, egg, water and margarine in mixing bowl. Beat until smooth. Stir in remaining cake mix. Drop by teaspoonfuls onto ungreased cookie sheet. Press tops with flour-dipped fork. Bake at 375 °F (175 °C) for 8 to 10 minutes. Cool slightly, then remove from pan.

Yield: 24 cookies
Exchange, 1 cookie: ½ bread
1 fat
Calories, 1 cookie: 68

Buttermilk Oat Crisps

8-oz. box	no-sugar chocolate cake mix	226-g box
1 c.	oatmeal	250 mL
½ c.	buttermilk	125 mL
½ c.	margarine, melted	125 mL

Combine ingredients in mixing bowl. Stir until dry ingredients are just moistened. Knead dough on very lightly floured board until mixture is completely blended. Roll out ⅛-in. (3-mm) thick. Cut into 2 × 4-in. (5 × 10-cm) rectangular strips. Place on ungreased cookie sheet. Bake at 400 °F (200 °C) for 6 to 8 minutes.

Yield: 54 cookies
Exchange, 1 cookie: ⅛ bread
⅖ fat
Calories, 1 cookie: 34

Sour Cream Drops

8-oz. box	*no-sugar chocolate cake mix*	*226-g box*
1	*egg*	*1*
⅓ c.	*sour cream*	*90 mL*

Combine all ingredients; mix to blend thoroughly. Chill at least 4 hours. Drop by teaspoonfuls onto greased cookie sheet. Bake at 350 °F (175 °C) for 8 to 12 minutes. Cool slightly; remove from pan.

Yield: 24 cookies
Exchange, 1 cookie: ½ bread
⅔ fat
Calories, 1 cookie: 47

Hang-Bangs

8-oz. box	*no-sugar chocolate cake mix*	*226-g box*
2½ T.	*water*	*37 mL*
1 T.	*almond extract*	*15 mL*
36	*almond halves, toasted*	*36*

Combine cake mix, water and almond extract in bowl. Beat until thoroughly blended. Drop by teaspoonfuls onto greased cookie sheet. Press an almond half into top of each cookie. Bake at 350 °F (175 °C) for 8 to 10 minutes.

Yield: 60 cookies
Exchange, 2 cookies: ⅓ bread
⅔ fat
Calories, 2 cookies: 28

Truffles

7-oz. box	no-sugar white frosting mix	200-g box
2 T.	cocoa	30 mL
2	egg yolks	2
1 T.	brandy flavoring	15 mL

Beat egg yolks until light and slightly thick. Add frosting mix, cocoa and brandy flavoring. Stir until completely blended. If needed, add water to make a workable paste. Shape dough into small balls. Place on waxed paper and let firm several hours in refrigerator.

Yield: 36 pieces
Exchange, 1 piece: ⅓ bread
½ fat
Calories, 1 piece: 38

Chocolate-Cherry Drops

8-oz. box	no-sugar chocolate cake mix	226-g box
1 T.	low-cal cherry preserves	15 mL
2 t.	cherry flavoring	10 mL
2 T.	water	30 mL

Combine all ingredients in mixing bowl; stir until completely blended. Drop by teaspoonfuls onto greased cookie sheet. Bake at 350 °F (175 °C) for 10 to 12 minutes.

Yield: 60 cookies
Exchange, 1 cookie: ⅓ bread
Calories, 1 cookie: 15

Pecan Balls

A real seller at church fairs.

8-oz. box	no-sugar chocolate cake mix	226-g box
1 T.	cornstarch	15 mL
¼ c.	pecans, finely ground	60 mL
3 T.	water	45 mL

Combine all ingredients in mixing bowl and stir to blend thoroughly. Cover bowl tightly; chill until firm. Roll in your palms into small, marble-size balls. Place on ungreased cookie sheet. Bake at 350 °F (175 °C) for 10 to 12 minutes.

Yield: 40 cookies
Exchange, 1 cookie: ⅓ bread
⅓ fat
Calories, 1 cookie: 31

Pineapple Queens

4½	sweet cherries	4½
8-oz. box	no-sugar chocolate cake mix	226-g box
¼ c.	crushed pineapple and unsweetened juice	60 mL

Drain cherries and pat dry. Cut each cherry into 8 slices, a total of 36 slices. In mixing bowl, combine cake mix and pineapple with its own juice. Stir to completely blend. Drop by teaspoonfuls onto greased cookie sheet. Top each cookie with a cherry slice. Bake at 350 °F (175 °C) for 10 to 12 minutes.

Yield: 36 cookies
Exchange, 1 cookie: ⅓ bread
Calories, 1 cookie: 26

Brownies and Bars

Chocolate-Mint Brownies

1 c.	flour	250 mL
½ t.	baking powder	2 mL
¼ t.	salt	1 mL
½ c.	vegetable shortening, softened	125 mL
½ c.	granulated sugar replacement	125 mL
3 T.	fructose	45 mL
3	eggs	3
2 oz.	baking chocolate, melted	60 g
1 T.	mint flavoring	15 mL
⅔ c.	no-sugar white frosting mix	165 mL
	green food coloring	
	hot water	
1 T.	chocolate sprinkles or jimmies	15 mL

Sift flour, baking powder and salt together. Cream shortening, sugar replacement and fructose; beat in eggs, melted chocolate and mint flavoring. Spread batter in two 8-in. (20-cm) greased pans. Bake at 325 °F (165 °C) for 25 to 30 minutes. Cool. Combine no-sugar frosting mix with a few drops of green food coloring and enough hot water to make frosting soft enough to spread. Spread on brownies; sprinkle tops with chocolate sprinkles. Cut into 1 × 2-in. (2.5 × 5-cm) bars.

Yield: 64 bars
Exchange, 1 bar: ⅓ bread
¾ fat
Calories, 1 bar: 41

Chocolate Pudding Brownies

⅓ c.	margarine, melted	90 mL
1 pkg.	reduced-calorie chocolate pudding mix	1 pkg.
2	eggs	2
1 t.	vanilla	15 mL
3 T.	water	45 mL
½ c.	flour	125 mL
¼ t.	baking powder	2 mL
⅓ c.	walnuts	90 mL

In medium-size bowl, combine margarine, pudding mix, eggs, vanilla and water. Beat to thoroughly mix. Add sifted flour and baking powder; stir until well blended. Fold in walnuts. Spread evenly into a greased 8-in. (20-cm) square pan. Bake at 350 °F (175 °C) for 15 minutes or until done. Cut into 2-in. (5-cm) squares.

Yield: 16 brownies
Exchange, 1 brownie: ½ bread
1 fat
Calories, 1 brownie: 78

Butterscotch-Chocolate Brownies

½ c.	margarine, melted	125 mL
1 env.	reduced-calorie butterscotch pudding mix	1 env.
1 env.	reduced-calorie chocolate pudding mix	1 env.
2	eggs	2
2 t.	vanilla	10 mL
⅓ c.	water	90 mL
1 c.	cake flour, sifted	250 mL
1½ t.	baking powder	7 mL

Combine margarine, pudding mixes, eggs, vanilla and water in medium size bowl; beat to blend thoroughly. Add cake flour and baking powder and continue beating until smooth and creamy. Pour into greased 8-in. (20-cm) square pan. Bake at 350 °F (175 °C) for 20 minutes or until done. Cut into 2-in. (5-cm) squares.

Yield: 16 brownies
Exchange, 1 brownie: ⅔ bread
1½ fat
Calories, 1 brownie: 94

Walnut Cubes

Crust

¾ c.	flour	250 mL
¼ c.	cocoa	60 mL
2 T.	granulated sugar replacement	30 mL
½ c.	butter	125 mL

Center Filling

2	eggs, well beaten	2
½ c.	granulated sugar replacement	125 mL
½ c.	unsweetened coconut, grated	125 mL
½ c.	walnuts, chopped	125 mL
2 T.	flour	30 mL
¼ t.	baking powder	1 mL
½ t.	salt	2 mL
1 t.	vanilla extract	5 mL

Frosting

1 c.	Powdered Sugar Replacement	250 mL
3 T.	cocoa	45 mL
2 T.	butter, melted	30 mL
2 T.	orange juice	30 mL
1 t.	orange rind, grated	5 mL
	water	

Combine flour, cocoa and granulated sugar replacement; work in the butter. Spread mixture in the bottom of a greased 9-in. (23-cm) pan. Bake at 350 °F (175 °C) for 15 minutes.

Combine center filling ingredients and stir to completely mix. Spread over crust. Return to oven and bake 25 minutes longer. Cool slightly.

Combine frosting ingredients and enough water to make a thick spreading paste, then spread on top of warm filling. Cool. Cut into 1-in. (2.5-cm) squares.

Yield: 81 cubes
Exchange, 2 cubes: ⅓ bread
1 fat
Calories, 2 cubes: 80

Hawaiian Coconut Bars

Crust

1 c.	flour, sifted	250 mL
3 T.	granulated brown sugar replacement	45 mL
¼ t.	salt	1 mL
¼ c.	margarine	60 mL
1 T.	water	15 mL

Topping

½ c.	flour	125 mL
½ t.	baking powder	2 mL
dash	salt	dash
1	egg	1
½ c.	granulated brown sugar replacement	125 mL
¼ c.	sorbitol	60 mL
1 T.	vanilla extract	15 mL
½ c.	mini chocolate chips	125 mL
½ c.	unsweetened coconut, shredded	125 mL
½ c.	unsweetened pineapple, crushed and well drained	125 mL

To prepare crust, blend flour, brown sugar and salt together, then cut in margarine. Work in water. Press into bottom of greased 13 × 9-in. (33 × 23-cm) pan. Bake at 350 °F (175 °C) for 10 minutes or until lightly browned.

To prepare topping, sift together the flour, baking powder and salt. Beat egg; gradually add brown sugar replacement and sorbitol. Add flour mixture, vanilla, mini chocolate chips, coconut and pineapple. Spread on top of crust. Bake at 350 °F (175 °C) for 35 to 40 minutes or until mixture is set. Cool slightly, cut into 1 × 3-in. (2.5 × 7.5-cm) bars.

Yield: 39 bars
Exchange, 1 bar: ⅓ bread
½ fat
Calories, 1 bar: 46

Delight Bar Cookies

1¾ c.	flour	440 mL
1 t.	baking powder	5 mL
½ t.	cloves, ground	2 mL
⅓ c.	cocoa	90 mL
⅓ c.	granulated brown sugar replacement	90 mL
¼ c.	sorbitol	60 mL
4	eggs, well beaten	4
1 c.	dried apricots, finely chopped	250 mL
¼ c.	walnuts, chopped	60 mL
	Powdered Sugar Replacement	

Sift flour, baking powder, cloves and cocoa together. Gradually, beat brown sugar replacement and sorbitol into eggs. Add dry ingredients. Fold in apricots and walnuts. Spread in three, greased 9-in. (23-cm) square pans. Bake at 350 °F (175 °C) for 25 to 30 minutes. Dust lightly with powdered sugar replacement. Cut into 1 × 3-in. (2.5 × 7.5-cm) bars.

Yield: 81 bars
Exchange, 1 bar: ⅕ bread
⅕ fat
Calories, 1 bar: 20

Frosted Coffee Creams

½ c.	vegetable shortening	125 mL
¼ c.	granulated brown sugar replacement	60 mL
¼ c.	granulated sugar replacement	60 mL
1 oz.	baking chocolate, melted	30 g
2	eggs	2
1½ c.	flour	375 mL
¼ t.	salt	1 mL
½ t.	baking soda	2 mL
½ t.	baking powder	2 mL
½ t.	nutmeg	2 mL
½ c.	cold strong coffee	125 mL
½ t.	vanilla extract	2 mL
7 oz.-pkg.	no-sugar white frosting mix	198-g pkg.
¼ c.	hot coffee	60 mL

Cream shortening; add sugar replacements and continue beating. Beat in melted chocolate and eggs until fluffy. Sift together flour, salt, baking soda, baking powder and nutmeg. Add to creamed mixture alternately with cold coffee. Add vanilla extract. Spread in greased 15½ × 10½-in. (39 × 25-cm) pan. Bake at 350 °F (175 °C) 20 to 25 minutes. Cool. Pour frosting mix into mixing bowl; gradually add hot coffee. Beat until smooth. Spread on cooled dough. Cut into 1½-in. (4-cm) squares.

Yield: 70 squares
Exchange, 1 square: ⅓ bread
                         ¾ fat
Calories, 1 square: 43

Afternoon Tea Brownies

1 c.	cake flour	250 mL
½ t.	salt	2 mL
1 t.	baking powder	5 mL
2 T.	cocoa	30 mL
1 oz.	baking chocolate, melted	30 g
¼ c.	vegetable shortening	60 mL
3	eggs	3
½ c.	granulated sugar replacement	125 mL
½ c.	skim milk	125 mL
½ c.	pecans, toasted and ground	125 mSL

Sift flour, salt, baking powder and cocoa together . Pour melted chocolate over shortening and stir until completely blended. Beat eggs until thick and lemon-colored; gradually add sugar replacement. Add chocolate mixture and small amount of flour mixture. Beat to thoroughly blend. Add remaining flour mixture alternately with the milk. Fold in the pecans. Spread in two 8-in. (20-cm) greased and paper-lined pans. Bake at 325 °F (165 °C) for 17 to 20 minutes. Cut into 1 × 2-in. (2.5 × 5-cm) bars.

Yield: 64 bars
Exchange, 2 bars: ⅓ bread
                        1 fat
Calories, 2 bars: 54

Fast-and-Easy Brownies

Fast-and-easy **anything** is great.

1 oz.	baking chocolate	30 g
⅓ c.	vegetable oil	90 mL
½ c.	granulated sugar replacement	125 mL
2	eggs	2
1 t.	vanilla extract	5 mL
¾ c.	cake flour, sifted	190 mL
½ t.	baking powder	2 mL
¼ t.	salt	1 mL

In top of double boiler, melt chocolate with oil. Remove from heat and beat in sugar replacement, eggs and vanilla extract. Stir in flour, baking powder and salt until well blended. Pour batter into well-greased 8-in. (20-cm) square pan. Bake at 350 °F (175 °C) for 25 to 30 minutes. Cut into 2-in. (5-cm) squares.

Yield: 16 brownies
Exchange, 1 brownie: ⅓ bread
1 fat
Calories, 1 brownie: 77

Basic Brownies

½ t.	baking powder	2 mL
½ t.	salt	2 mL
3 oz.	unsweetened chocolate, melted	90 g
½ c.	shortening, softened	125 mL
2	eggs	2
2 T.	granulated sugar replacement	30 mL
1½ c.	flour	375 mL
1 t.	vanilla extract	5 mL

Combine all ingredients and beat vigorously until well blended. Spread mixture into greased 8-in. (20-cm) square pan. Bake at 350 °F (175 °C) for 30 to 35 minutes. Cut into 2-in. (5-cm) squares.
Microwave: Cook on medium for 8 to 10 minutes or until puffed and dry on top. Cut into 2-in. (5-cm) squares.

Yield: 16 brownies
Exchange, 1 brownie: 1½ bread
1½ fat
Calories, 1 brownie: 136

Black 'n' White Brownies

A college favorite—these brownies are mailable.

1 c.	cake flour	250 mL
1 t.	baking powder	5 mL
¼ t.	salt	1 mL
½ c.	shortening, softened	125 mL
½ c.	granulated sugar replacement	125 mL
2	eggs	2
1 t.	vanilla extract	5 mL
1 T.	water	15 mL
¼ c.	unsweetened coconut, grated	60 mL
1 t.	coconut milk	5 mL
1 oz.	baking chocolate, melted	30 g

Sift together the flour, baking powder and salt. Cream shortening and sugar replacement until light and fluffy. Add eggs, one at a time, beating well after each addition. Beat in vanilla extract and water. Divide batter into two equal parts. To one part add unsweetened coconut and coconut milk. Stir to completely blend. To the remaining half, beat in the melted chocolate. Spread coconut mixture on bottom of well-greased 8-in. (20-cm) square pan. Spread chocolate layer on top of coconut layer. Bake at 350 °F (175 °C) for 25 to 30 minutes. Cut into 1 × 2-in. (2.5 × 5-cm) bars.

Yield: 32 bars
Exchange, 1 bar: ⅓ bread
1 fat
Calories, 1 bar: 54

Chocolate Yum-Yums

½ c.	vegetable shortening	125 mL
2 oz.	baking chocolate	60 g
½ c.	granulated brown sugar replacement	125 mL
2 T.	fructose	30 mL
1	egg, well beaten	1
2 T.	water	30 mL
1½ c.	flour	375 mL
½ t.	baking soda	2 mL
dash	salt	dash
½ c.	skim milk	125 mL
1 t.	vanilla extract	5 mL
¼ c.	brazil nuts, finely chopped	60 mL
¼ c.	unsweetened coconut, grated	60 mL

Melt shortening and baking chocolate; add brown sugar replacement and fructose, stir until smooth. Cool. Add egg and water and mix thoroughly. Sift dry ingredients together. Add dry ingredients alternately with milk and vanilla extract. Pour into a 15½ × 10 ½-in. (39 × 25-cm) greased jelly roll pan. Sprinkle with chopped brazil nuts and coconut. Bake at 350 °F (175 °C) for 10 to 12 minutes. Cool slightly and cut into 1½-in. (4-cm) squares.

Yield: 70 squares
Exchange, 1 square: ⅓ bread
1 fat
Calories, 1 square: 36

Peanut Sticks

2	eggs, well beaten	2
½ c.	granulated sugar replacement	125 mL
2 T.	fructose	30 mL
1 T.	margarine	30 mL
1 oz.	baking chocolate, melted	30 g
½ c.	skim milk, boiling	125 mL
1½ c.	flour, sifted	375 mL
2 t.	baking powder	10 mL
7-oz. pkg.	no-sugar chocolate frosting mix	198-g pkg.
1 c.	peanuts, finely ground	250 mL

Blend together the eggs, sugar replacement, fructose, margarine and baking chocolate. Add skim milk and stir until smooth. Add flour and baking powder. Stir to completely blend. Divide batter into two greased 8-in. (20-cm) square cake pans. Bake at 375 °F (190 °C) for 20 to 25 minutes. Cool. Make frosting as directed on package; add peanuts. Spread frosting on cooled dough. Cut into 1 × 2-in. (2.5 × 5-cm) sticks.

Yield: 64 sticks
Exchange, 1 stick: ⅓ bread
1 fat
Calories, 1 stick: 49

Goodlies

The name for this treat is an inside joke. In our home, whenever we taste foods that everyone likes, we call them "goodlies." Ages 8 to 80 love them.

1 c.	cake flour	250 mL
⅓ c.	granulated sugar replacement	90 mL
2½ c.	oatmeal	625 mL
1 c.	margarine, softened	250 mL
¾ c.	Chocolate Topping	190 mL

Combine cake flour, sugar replacement and oatmeal in a bowl; cut in margarine until all ingredients are blended into a crumbly dough. Press one-half of the dough into the bottom of a 11 × 7-in. (27 × 17-cm) well-greased pan. Spread ½ c. (125 mL) of the chocolate topping over the entire surface. Sprinkle with remaining dough and gently press the top dough. Drizzle with remaining chocolate topping. Bake at 350 °F (175 °C) for 25 to 30 minutes. Cool slightly. Cut into 1-in. (2.5-cm) squares.

Yield: 77 squares
Exchange, 1 square: ⅓ bread
½ fat
Calories, 1 square: 32

Date Brownies

¾ c.	cake flour	190 mL
½ t.	baking powder	2 mL
dash	salt	dash
½ c.	dates, finely chopped	125 mL
½ c.	vegetable shortening, softened	125 mL
½ c.	granulated sugar replacement	125 mL
2	eggs	2
2 t.	vanilla extract	10 mL
1 oz.	baking chocolate, melted	30 g
	Powdered Sugar Replacement	

Sift flour, baking powder and salt together. Stir chopped dates into flour mixture. Cream shortening and gradually add sugar replacement. Beat until light and fluffy. Continue beating and add eggs and vanilla extract. Beat in chocolate. Stir in flour/date mixture. Spread evenly in a greased 8-in. (20-cm) pan. Bake at 350 °F (175 °C) for 25 to 30 minutes. Cool and dust lightly with powdered sugar replacement. Cut into 1 × 2-in. (2.5 × 5-cm) bars.

Yield: 32 bars
Exchange, 1 bar: ⅓ bread
1 fat
Calories, 1 bar: 54

Pineapple-Nut Brownies

These brownies seem to appeal to men.

1 c.	flour	250 mL
½ t.	baking powder	2 mL
¼ t.	baking soda	1 mL
¼ t.	salt	1 mL
½ c.	margarine	125 mL
1 oz.	baking chocolate	30 g
½ c.	granulated sugar replacement	125 mL
2	eggs, beaten	2
8-oz. can	crushed, canned pineapple, drained	227-g can
1 t.	almond extract	5 mL
⅓ c.	walnuts, chopped	90 mL

Sift flour, baking powder, baking soda and salt together. In the top of a double boiler, melt margarine and baking chocolate; blend in sugar replacement. Remove from heat. Beat in eggs, pineapple and almond extract. Stir in flour mixture until well blended. Fold in walnuts. Pour into a greased 8-in. (20-cm) square pan. Bake at 350 °F (175 °C) for 30 to 35 minutes. Cool and cut into 1 × 2-in (2.5 × 5-cm) bars.

Yield: 32 bars
Exchange, 1 bar: ⅓ bread
          1 fat
Calories, 1 bar: 60

English Toffee Squares

A sweet and nutty taste.

1 t.	salt	5 mL
1 t.	cinnamon	5 mL
2 c.	cake flour	500 mL
¾ c.	butter	190 mL
½ c.	granulated sugar replacement	125 mL
1 oz.	baking chocolate, melted	30 g
1	egg yolk	1
2 t.	vanilla extract	10 mL
½ c.	pecans, finely chopped	125 mL
1	egg white	1

Sift together salt, cinnamon and flour. Cream butter and sugar replacement. Beat in baking chocolate and egg yolk. Add sifted dry ingredients and mix. Add vanilla extract and pecans. Mix well, press dough into a greased 14 × 10-in. (35 × 25-cm) cookie sheet. Beat egg white until frothy. Spread egg white over dough in pan. Bake at 375 °F (190 °C) for 25 minutes. Cut into 2-in. (5-cm) squares.

Yield: 35 squares
Exchange, 1 square: ⅓ bread
              1 fat
Calories, 1 square: 74

Chocolate Chiefs

2	eggs	2
½ c.	granulated sugar replacement	125 mL
1 t.	vanilla extract	5 mL
¼ c.	skim milk	60 mL
2 oz.	baking chocolate, melted	60 g
dash	salt	dash
1 c.	cake flour	250 mL
⅓ c.	hazelnuts, coarsely chopped	90 mL

Beat eggs until thick and lemon-colored. Gradually add sugar replacement. Beat in vanilla extract and skim milk. Add the melted chocolate, salt, flour and hazelnuts. Spread in well-greased, paper-lined 11 × 7-in. (27 × 17-cm) pan. Bake at 350 °F (175 °C) for 25 to 30 minutes. Remove from pan and cut into 1-in. (2.5-cm) squares.

Yield: 77 squares
Exchange, 2 squares: ⅕ bread
                     ⅕ fat
Calories, 2 squares: 29

Quick Brownies and Bars

Black Forest Bars

Who says "Black Forest" is a cake?

16-oz. can	sour cherries, pitted	454-g can
8-oz. pkg.	no-sugar chocolate cake mix	266-g pkg.
2 T.	granulated sugar replacement	30 mL

Drain cherries very well. Combine cake mix, cherries and sugar replacement in mixing bowl. Stir to blend thoroughly. Spread batter in well-greased 9-in. (23-cm) pan. Bake at 375 °F (190 °C) for 20 to 25 minutes. Cut into 1 × 1½-in. (2.5 × 4-cm) bars.

Yield: 54 bars
Exchange, 1 bar: ¼ bread
Calories, 1 bar: 20

Blond Brownies

8-oz. pkg.	no-sugar white cake mix	226-g pkg.
2	eggs	2
2 T.	granulated brown sugar replacement	30 mL
2 T.	water	30 mL
¼ c.	mini chocolate chips	60 mL
¼ c.	peanut butter chips	60 mL

Combine cake mix, eggs, brown sugar replacement and water in mixing bowl. Beat at medium speed until well blended and thickened. Fold in chips. Pour batter into two, greased and papered 8-in. (20-cm) pans. Bake at 375 °F (190 °C) for 12 to 15 minutes or until brownies test done. Cut into 2-in. (5-cm) squares.

Yield: 32 squares
Exchange, 1 square: ⅓ bread
                            ½ fat
Calories, 1 square: 56

Pistachio Bars

LOVE those pistachio nuts!

8-oz. box	sugar-restricted chocolate cake mix	226-g box
⅓ c.	hot water	90 mL
⅓ c.	pistachio nuts, finely chopped	90 mL

Combine all ingredients and stir to completely blend. Spread batter evenly in a greased and papered 8-in. (20-cm) pan. Bake at 350 °F (175 °C) for 20 to 25 minutes. Cool slightly; cut into 1-in. (2.5-cm) squares.

Yield: 32 squares
Exchange, 1 square: ⅓ bread
                            ⅓ fat
Calories, 1 square: 35

Delicious Cakes

Spragg Cake

Dedicated to W. Spragg, a diligent helper in the diabetes work being done in Iowa. This is yours, Mr. Spragg.

¼ c.	almonds, toasted and ground	60 mL
½ c.	semisweet chocolate chips	125 mL
2 T.	butter	30 mL
¼ c.	skim milk	60 mL
5	egg yolks	5
5 T.	cornstarch	75 mL
4 T.	granulated sugar replacement	60 mL
1 T.	almond extract	15 mL
1 t.	instant coffee	5 mL
1 T.	flour	15 mL
5	egg whites	5

Combine ground almonds, chocolate chips, butter and milk in saucepan. Cook and stir over low heat until chocolate is melted; cool. Beat egg yolks with an electric mixer on high speed until pale yellow, gradually adding 3 T. (45 mL) of the cornstarch and 2 T. (30 mL) of the sugar replacement. Add egg yolk mixture to cooled chocolate mixture. Fold in almond extract, coffee and flour. In another bowl, with clean beaters beat egg whites until stiff. Gradually add remaining 2 T. (30 mL) cornstarch and 2 T. (30 mL) sugar replacement. Gently fold a large spoonful of whites into chocolate mixture to lighten, then fold remaining whites into chocolate mixture. Pour batter into well-greased 10-in. (25-cm) springform pan. Bake at top of 350 °F (175 °C) oven for 40 to 50 minutes or until cake springs back when lightly touched.

Yield: 20 servings
Exchange, 1 serving: ½ bread
1 fat
Calories, 1 serving: 69

Chocolate Cake

1½ c.	flour	375 mL
¼ c.	granulated sugar replacement	60 mL
½ c.	unsweetened cocoa	125 mL
1½ t.	baking soda	7 mL
1 t.	salt	5 mL
1 c.	low-fat milk (2% milk fat)	250 mL
⅔ c.	vegetable oil	180 mL
2	eggs	2

Combine all ingredients in large bowl and beat just until blended. Pour into well-greased and floured 13 × 9-in. (33 × 23-cm) cake pan. Bake at 350 °F (175 °C) for 40 to 45 minutes, or until done.

Yield: 24 servings
Exchange, 1 serving: ½ bread
1 fat
Calories, 1 serving: 86

D.C.N. Pudding Cake

D.C.N. stands for dates, chips and nuts.

3	eggs	3
3 T.	granulated sugar replacement	45 mL
¼ c.	flour	60 mL
1 t.	baking powder	5 mL
¼ t.	salt	1 mL
½ c.	dates, finely chopped	125 mL
⅓ c.	mini chocolate chips	90 mL
¼ c.	walnuts, finely chopped	60 mL

Beat eggs in large mixing bowl until light and fluffy. Gradually add sugar replacement, beating continually until thick. Stir in flour, baking powder and salt. Mix in dates, chocolate chips and nuts. Pour batter into well-greased 9-in. (23-cm) square baking pan. Bake at 350 °F (175 °C) for 25 to 30 minutes or until cake tests done. Serve warm.

Yield: 9 servings
Exchange, 1 serving: 1 bread
1¼ fat
Calories, 1 serving: 118

Brownie Cake

⅓ c.	butter	90 mL
¼ c.	granulated sugar replacement	60 mL
4	eggs	4
3 T.	Chocolate Syrup	45 mL
1 c.	flour	250 mL
1 t.	baking powder	5 mL
dash	salt	dash
1½ t.	vanilla extract	7 mL
½ recipe	Marshmallow Crème	½ recipe
1 recipe	Chocolate Drizzle	1 recipe

Cream butter with sugar replacement until fluffy. Add eggs and beat well. Stir in chocolate syrup. Sift flour, baking powder and salt into small bowl. Blend flour mixture into chocolate mixture. Add vanilla extract. Pour batter into well-greased, 9 × 13-in. (23 × 33-cm) baking pan. Bake at 350 °F (175 °C) for 30 to 40 minutes or until cake tests done. Cool. Cover cake with marshmallow crème, then the chocolate drizzle.

Yield: 24 servings
Exchange, 1 serving: ½ bread
1 fat
Calories, 1 serving: 63

Rum Roll

An **extra-special** cake with few calories.

¾ c.	cake flour	190 mL
1 t.	baking powder	5 mL
½ t.	baking soda	2 mL
dash	salt	dash
3	egg whites	3
1 T.	white vinegar	15 mL
1 T.	water	15 mL
¼ c.	semisweet chocolate chips	60 mL
3 T.	sorbitol	45 mL
3 T.	granulated sugar replacement	45 mL
⅓ c.	water, boiling	90 mL
3	egg yolks	3
2 T.	rum flavoring	30 mL
1 t.	vanilla extract	5 mL
1 recipe	Chocolate Whipped Topping	1 recipe

Sift together 3 times the cake flour, baking powder, baking soda and salt. Whip egg whites until soft peaks form; gradually, add vinegar and water and continue whipping into stiff peaks. In a bowl combine chocolate chips, sorbitol, and sugar replacement. Add boiling water and stir until chocolate is melted. Add egg yolks, rum and vanilla extract. Beat until smooth and slightly fluffy. Fold in dry flour mixture. Fold in egg whites. Do not over mix; some streaks of egg white may remain. Gently, spread mixture into papered, well-greased and floured jelly roll pan. Bake at 325 °F (165 °C) for 13 to 15 minutes or until cake tests done. Invert cake onto a lightly floured pastry towel or cloth. Peel off paper. Gently roll up cake and towel. Place on cooling rack and allow to cool. Unroll cake, spread with the chocolate whipped topping. Roll up without squeezing whipped topping from cake. Chill in refrigerator or freeze.

Yield: 24 servings
Exchange, 1 serving: ½ bread
Calories, 1 serving: 29

Fudge Cupcakes

½ c.	butter	125 mL
3 oz.	baking chocolate	90 g
½ c.	granulated sugar replacement	125 mL
2 c.	flour	500 mL
dash	salt	dash
8	eggs, lightly beaten	8
1 T.	vanilla extract	15 mL

Melt butter with chocolate in top of double boiler over warm water. In large mixing bowl combine sugar replacement, flour and salt; stir in melted chocolate mixture. Add eggs and vanilla extract. Stir just until moistened and blended. Spoon batter into muffin pans lined with paper muffin cups. Bake muffins at 300 °F (150 °C) for 35 minutes or until muffins test done.

Yield: 36 muffins
Exchange, 1 muffin: ½ bread
1 fat
Calories, 1 muffin: 78

Muse Cake

1 medium	orange with rind	1 medium
½ c.	raisins	125 mL
2 c.	flour	500 mL
¼ c.	granulated fructose	60 mL
3 T.	granulated sugar replacement	45 mL
1 oz.	baking chocolate, melted	30 g
¾ c.	buttermilk	190 mL
2	eggs	2
2 T.	butter, softened	30 mL
1 t.	baking soda	5 mL
¼ t.	salt	1 mL

Squeeze juice from orange and set aside. Chop orange rind into small pieces. Combine chopped rind, raisins and 2 T. (30 mL) of the flour in blender. Blend until finely chopped. Transfer to large mixing bowl. Add remaining flour, fructose, sugar replacement, melted chocolate, buttermilk, eggs, butter, baking soda and salt. Stir to completely blend. Pour batter into well-greased, 9 × 13-in. (23 × 33-cm) baking pan. Bake at 350 °F (175 °C) for 40 to 50 minutes or until cake tests done. Remove from oven; immediately pour reserved orange juice over entire surface.

Yield: 24 servings
Exchange, 1 serving: ¾ bread
½ fat
Calories, 1 serving: 75

Chocolate Walnut-Filled Cake

Cake

2 c.	cake flour	500 mL
½ c.	cocoa	125 mL
3 T.	granulated sugar replacement	45 mL
1 T.	baking powder	15 mL
1¼ c.	milk	310 mL
¼ c.	margarine, softened	60 mL
2	eggs	2

Combine cake flour, cocoa, sugar replacement and baking powder in sifter. Sift into medium bowl, add remaining ingredients and beat until smooth and creamy. Pour into well-greased and floured 3-qt. (3-L) fluted tube pan.

Filling

½ c.	all-purpose flour	125 mL
⅓ c.	walnuts, very finely chopped	90 mL
⅓ c.	milk	90 mL
1 t.	granulated sugar replacement	5 mL
1 t.	baking powder	5 mL
1 t.	vanilla extract	5 mL

Combine all ingredients in small bowl, mixing with fork until well blended. Spoon in a ring over center of chocolate batter (above), but do not touch sides of pan with filling. Bake at 350 °F (175 °C) for 35 minutes or until done. Cool in pan 20 to 25 minutes, invert onto cooling rack or plate and cool completely. Frost with favorite glaze.

Yield: 24 servings
Exchange, 1 serving: ⅔ bread
½ lean meat
Calories, 1 serving: 84

Peppermint Cake

2 c.	cake flour, sifted	500 mL
1 t.	baking soda	5 mL
½ t.	salt	2 mL
⅓ c.	vegetable shortening, softened	90 mL
¼ c.	granulated sugar replacement	60 mL
1	egg	1
2 oz.	baking chocolate, melted	60 g
½ t.	peppermint oil	2 mL
2 t.	vanilla extract	10 mL
½ c.	unflavored yogurt	125 mL
¾ c.	skim milk	190 mL

Sift flour, baking soda and salt together. Cream shortening and sugar replacement until light and fluffy. Add egg and beat well. Add chocolate, peppermint oil and vanilla and blend thoroughly. Beat in yogurt. Add flour mixture and milk alternately in small amounts; beat well after each addition. Pour batter into two well-greased 9-in. (23-cm) pans or one 9 × 13-in. (23 × 33-cm) pan. Bake at 350 °F (175 °C) for 30 to 40 minutes or until cake tests done.

Yield: 24 servings
Exchange, 1 serving: ½ bread
1 fat
Calories, 1 serving: 82

Mint Chip Cake

1½ c.	cake flour, sifted	375 mL
2 t.	baking powder	10 mL
dash	salt	dash
½ c.	shortening	125 mL
¼ c.	granulated sugar replacement	60 mL
½ c.	skim milk	125 mL
3	eggs, separated	3
¼ c.	fructose	60 mL
1½ t.	vanilla extract	7 mL
2 t.	mint flavoring	10 mL
¼ c.	mini chocolate chips	60 g

Sift flour, baking powder and salt together. Cream shortening with sugar replacement until fluffy. Beat egg yolks until thick; add fructose and continue beating until very thick. Add to shortening mixture. Add sifted dry ingredients and milk alternately in small amounts; beat well after each addition. Beat egg whites until stiff. Fold egg whites, vanilla extract, mint flavoring and chocolate chips into batter. Pour into two 8-in. (20-cm) well-greased and floured pans. Bake at 350 °F (175 °C) for 25 to 30 minutes or until cake tests done.

Yield: 18 servings
Exchange, 1 serving: ¾ bread
1½ fat
Calories, 1 serving: 109

German Chocolate Cake

A choice for all birthdays.

4 oz.	baking chocolate	120 g
½ c.	water, boiling	125 mL
½ c.	butter	125 mL
½ c.	granulated sugar replacement	125 mL
3 T.	granulated fructose	45 mL
4	egg yolks	4
2 t.	vanilla extract	10 mL
2¼ c.	flour	625 mL
1 t.	baking soda	5 mL
½ t.	salt	2 mL
1 c.	buttermilk	250 mL
4	egg whites, stiffly beaten	4

Melt chocolate in boiling water. Cool. Cream butter, sugar replacement and fructose until fluffy. Add egg yolks, one at a time, beating well after each addition. Blend in vanilla and chocolate water. Sift flour with baking soda and salt; add alternately with buttermilk to chocolate mixture, beating well after each addition until smooth. Fold in beaten egg whites. Grease three 9-in. (23-cm) baking pans and line them with paper; grease again and lightly flour pans; pour batter into the three pans. Bake at 350 °F (175 °C) for 25 to 30 minutes or until cakes test done. Remove from pans onto racks, remove paper lining. Cool.

Yield: three 9-in. (23-cm) cakes or 60 servings
Exchange, 1 serving: ½ bread
½ fat
Calories, 1 serving: 50

Pioneer Chocolate Cake

3 c.	flour	750 mL
¼ t.	salt	1 mL
1 t.	baking soda	5 mL
1 pkg.	dry yeast	1 pkg.
½ c.	warm water	125 mL
½ c.	shortening, softened	125 mL
½ c.	granulated sugar replacement	125 mL
3 T.	sorbitol	45 mL
3	eggs	3
1 c.	skim milk	250 mL
2 oz.	baking chocolate, melted	60 g
⅓ c.	walnuts, chopped	90 mL

Sift flour, salt and baking soda together. Soften yeast in warm water; set aside until swollen. Cream shortening, sugar replacement and sorbitol until light and fluffy. Add eggs, one at a time, beating well after each addition. Beat in swollen yeast. Add milk, chocolate, dry ingredients and nuts. Beat for 5 to 7 minutes or until mixture is fairly thick. Pour into well-greased 9 × 13-in. (23 × 33-cm) pan. Cover with waxed paper and light cloth. Place in warm, draft-free place to rise for one hour; or place in refrigerator for 6 hours or overnight. Bake at 350 °F (175 °C) for 45 minutes or until cake tests done.

Yield: 24 servings
Exchange, 1 serving: 1 bread
1½ fat
Calories, 1 serving: 129

Banana Chocolate Cake

2¼ c.	cake flour	560 mL
1 t.	baking powder	5 mL
1 t.	baking soda	5 mL
1 t.	salt	5 mL
⅔ c.	shortening, softened	165 mL
½ c.	granulated sugar replacement	125 mL
2	eggs	2
2 oz.	baking chocolate, melted	60 g
1 t.	vanilla extract	5 mL
3	bananas, mashed	3
½ c.	buttermilk	125 mL

Sift flour, baking powder, baking soda and salt together. Cream shortening with sugar replacement until fluffy. Add eggs, one at a time; beat well after each addition. Add chocolate and mix thoroughly. Stir in vanilla extract. Add dry ingredients alternately with mashed bananas and milk in small amounts. Beat well after each addition. Pour into two well-greased and floured 9-in. (23-cm) pans. Bake at 350 °F (175 °C) for 30 to 35 minutes or until cake tests done.

Yield: 24 servings
Exchange, 1 serving: 1 bread
1½ fat
Calories, 1 serving: 118

Cheese 'n' Chip Cake

8 oz.	cream cheese, softened	226 g
⅓ c.	butter, softened	90 mL
⅓ c.	granulated fructose	90 mL
3 T.	granulated sugar replacement	45 mL
6	eggs	6
3 c.	cake flour	750 mL
⅓ c.	chocolate chips	90 mL
1 T.	vanilla extract	15 mL
1 t.	lemon extract	5 mL

Beat cream cheese and butter with fructose and sugar replacement until smooth. Add eggs, one at a time, alternately with flour, stirring well after each addition. Fold in chocolate chips and extract. Pour batter into a well-greased and floured 3 qt. (3 L) Bundt pan. Bake at 350 °F (175 °C) for 30 minutes. Reduce heat to 325 °F (165 °C) and bake about 35 to 45 minutes longer or until cake tests done. Cool in pan on rack.

Yield: 24 servings
Exchange, 1 serving: 1 bread
1½ fat
Calories, 1 serving: 121

Sour-Milk Chocolate Cake

A cake superlative.

2 c.	cake flour, sifted	500 mL
1 t.	baking soda	5 mL
¼ t.	salt	1 mL
½ c.	vegetable shortening, softened	125 mL
¼ c.	granulated sugar replacement	60 mL
2 t.	vanilla extract	10 mL
3	egg yolks, beaten	3
2 oz.	baking chocolate, melted	60 g
1 c.	skim milk, soured (see note below)	250 mL
3	egg whites, stiffly beaten	3

Sift flour, baking soda and salt together. Cream shortening and sugar replacement until fluffy; add vanilla extract and egg yolks and beat thoroughly. Stir in chocolate. Add sifted dry ingredients and soured milk alternately in small amounts; beat well after each addition. Fold in stiffly beaten egg whites. Pour batter into two 9-in. (23-cm) well greased and floured pans. Bake at 350 °F (175 °C) for 30 to 35 minutes or until cake tests done.

Note: To sour 1 c. (250 mL) milk, stir in 2 t. (10 mL) vinegar or lemon juice.

Yield: 24 servings (12 servings per cake)
Exchange, 1 serving: ½ bread
1¼ fat
Calories, 1 serving: 95

Marble Cake

Only for rare occasions.

1¾ c.	cake flour	440 mL
2¼ t.	baking powder	12 mL
¼ t.	salt	1 mL
½ c.	vegetable shortening, softened	125 mL
3 T.	granulated sugar replacement	45 mL
2	eggs, well beaten	2
½ c.	skim milk	125 mL
2 t.	vanilla extract	10 mL
1 oz.	baking chocolate, melted	30 g

Sift flour, baking powder and salt together. Cream shortening with sugar replacement until fluffy. Add beaten eggs and mix thoroughly. Add sifted dry ingredients and milk alternately in small amounts, beating well after each addition. Add vanilla extract. Divide batter into two equal parts. Add chocolate to one part of the batter. Drop batter alternately by tablespoons into well-greased 8-in. (20-cm) square baking pan. Bake at 350 °F (175 °C) for 45 to 55 minutes until cake tests done.

Yield: 9 servings
Exchange, 1 serving: 1 bread
3 fat
Calories, 1 serving: 218

Wacky Chocolate Cake

1½ c.	cake flour	375 mL
¼ c.	cocoa	60 mL
2 T.	granulated sugar replacement	30 mL
1 t.	baking soda	5 mL
½ t.	salt	2 mL
1 c.	water	250 mL
1 T.	white vinegar	15 mL
¼ c.	vegetable oil	60 mL
1 t.	vanilla extract	5 mL
1	egg	1

Combine cake flour, cocoa, sugar replacement, baking soda and salt in sifter. Sift into large bowl, add remaining ingredients and beat to mix. Pour into 9-in. (23-cm) square baking dish. Bake at 375 °F (190 °C) for 35 to 40 minutes, or until done.
Microwave: Cook on medium for 10 to 11 minutes, turning dish a quarter turn every 5 minutes.

Yield: 9 servings
Exchange, 1 serving: 1 bread
1 fat
Calories, 1 serving: 89

Cocoa Spice Cake

The spices make the difference.

2 c.	flour	500 mL
½ c.	cocoa	125 mL
¼ t.	salt	1 mL
1 t.	baking soda	5 mL
2 t.	cinnamon	10 mL
1 t.	cloves	5 mL
½ t.	nutmeg	2 mL
½ c.	vegetable shortening, softened	125 mL
¼ c.	granulated brown sugar replacement	60 mL
3	eggs, separated	3
1 c.	sour cream	250 mL

Sift together 3 times the flour, cocoa, salt, soda and spices. Cream shortening with brown sugar replacement until fluffy. Beat egg yolks thoroughly and add to batter. Add sifted dry ingredients and sour cream alternately in small amounts, beating well after each addition. Beat egg whites until stiff, but not dry, and fold into batter. Pour into greased 9-in. (23-cm) square pan. Bake at 350 °F (175 °C) for 40 to 50 minutes or until cake tests done.

Yield: 9 servings
Exchange, 1 serving: 1½ bread
3 fat
Calories, 1 serving: 242

Devil's Food Cake

2¼ c.	cake flour	560 mL
¼ c.	granulated sugar replacement	60 mL
2 t.	baking soda	10 mL
1 t.	salt	5 mL
½ c.	cocoa	125 mL
⅔ c.	vegetable shortening, softened	180 mL
1 c.	water	250 mL
2 t.	vanilla extract	10 mL
3	eggs	3

Sift flour, sugar replacement, baking soda, salt and cocoa together into large mixing bowl. Add shortening, ½ c. (125 mL) of the water and vanilla extract; beat until just moistened. Add remaining water and eggs. Beat until slightly thickened. Pour into well-greased and floured 13 × 9-in. (23 × 33-cm) baking pan. Bake at 350 °F (175 °C) for 40 to 50 minutes or until cake tests done.

Yield: 24 servings
Exchange, 1 serving: ½ bread
1½ fat
Calories, 1 serving: 99

Quick Cakes

Brandy Cake

8-oz. box	no-sugar chocolate cake mix	226-g box
½ c.	buttermilk	125 mL
1	egg	1
2 t.	brandy flavoring	10 mL

Combine all ingredients and blend with an electric mixer on medium speed for 4 minutes. Pour into an 8- or 9-in. (20- or 23-cm) baking pan. Bake at 350 °F (175 °C) for 25 to 30 minutes or until cake tests done.

Yield: 9 servings
Exchange, 1 serving: 1⅓ bread
⅗ fat
Calories, 1 serving: 112

Pumpkin Cake

8-oz. box	no-sugar chocolate cake mix	226-g box
1	egg	1
1/4 c.	water	60 mL
1 t.	baking soda	5 mL
1 c.	pumpkin purée	250 mL
1 t.	pumpkin pie spice	5 mL

Combine all ingredients and blend with an electric mixer on medium speed for 4 minutes. Pour into greased 8- or 9-in. (20- or 23-cm) baking pan. Bake at 350 °F (175 °C) for 25 to 30 minutes or until cake tests done.

Yield: 9 servings
Exchange, 1 serving: 1¼ bread
⅗ fat
Calories, 1 serving: 117

Cocoa Cake

3 T.	cocoa	45 mL
1½ c.	flour	375 mL
1/4 c.	granulated sugar replacement	60 mL
1 t.	baking soda	5 mL
1/2 t.	salt	2 mL
1/3 c.	liquid shortening	90 mL
1 T.	white vinegar	15 mL
1 T.	vanilla extract	15 mL
1 c.	water	250 mL

Combine all ingredients in large mixing bowl. Beat to blend thoroughly. Pour batter into 9-in. (23-cm) square baking pan. Bake at 350 °F (175 °C) for 20 to 30 minutes or until cake tests done. Serve warm.

Yield: 9 servings
Exchange, 1 serving: 1 bread
1½ fat
Calories, 1 serving: 149

Chocolate-Cherry Cake

A delicious cake for any occasion.

8-oz. box	*sugar-restricted chocolate cake mix*	226-g box
1 c.	*tart cherries, in their own juice*	250 mL
3 T.	*granulated sugar replacement*	45 mL

Combine all ingredients and stir to completely blend. Pour into a well-greased 8- or 9-in. (20- or 23-cm) baking pan. Bake at 350 °F (175 °C) for 30 to 35 minutes or until cake tests done.

Yield: 9 servings
Exchange, 1 serving: 1 bread
                          ½ fat
Calories, 1 serving: 100

Peanut Butter Cake

Chocolate and peanut butter made easy.

8-oz. box	*sugar-restricted chocolate cake mix*	226-g box
½ c.	*chunky peanut butter*	125 mL

Prepare cake mix as directed on package and add peanut butter. Bake at 375 °F (190 °C) for 25 minutes or until cake tests done.

Yield: 10 servings
Exchange, 1 serving: 1 bread
                          2 fat
Calories, 1 serving: 169

Perfect Pastries

Cream Puff Pastry

1 c.	water	250 mL
¼ c.	margarine	60 mL
dash	salt	dash
1 c.	flour	250 mL
4	eggs	4

Combine water, margarine and salt in medium saucepan. Cook and stir over high heat until boiling; reduce heat. Add flour and cook and stir over medium heat until mixture comes clean from sides of pan and forms ball in center. Remove from heat; cool slightly. With spoon, electric beater or food processor, add eggs, one at a time. Beat after each addition until batter is smooth and glossy. Follow directions below.

For cream puffs: Drop tablespoonfuls onto lightly greased baking sheets. Bake at 425 °F (220 °C) for 15 minutes; reduce heat to 350 °F (175 °C) and bake 25 minutes longer, or until puffs are free of moisture beads. (Puff pastry will collapse if removed from oven early.) Remove from oven. Remove tops or cut into sides to allow hot air to escape; cool completely.

For eclairs: Spoon pastry batter into pastry bag fitted with ½-in. (1.25-cm) tube. Shape batter into 1 × 4-in. (2 × 10-cm) strips. Bake as for cream puffs.

Yield: 10 puffs or eclairs
Exchange, 1 puff or eclair: ⅔ full-fat milk
Calories, 1 puff or eclair: 114

For Mini-Cream Puffs: Drop teaspoonfuls onto lightly greased baking sheets. Bake at 425 °F (220 °C) for 15 minutes; reduce heat to 350 °F (175 °C) and bake 25 minutes longer. Cut small hole in top; cool completely.

Yield: 30 puffs
Exchange, 1 puff: ⅓ bread
½ fat
Calories, 1 puff: 37

Mosaic Chocolate Torte

Enjoy every bite.

1 t.	unflavored gelatin	5 mL
1 T.	cold water	15 mL
2 oz.	baking chocolate	60 g
¼ c.	granulated sugar replacement	60 mL
2 T.	sorbitol	30 mL
dash	salt	dash
¼ c.	hot water	60 mL
4	eggs, separated	4
1 t.	vanilla extract	5 mL
1 c.	nondairy whipped topping	250 mL
½	Sponge Cake	½

Soften gelatin in cold water; set aside. Melt baking chocolate in top of double boiler. Add sugar replacement, sorbitol, salt and hot water. Stir until mixture is well blended. Add softened gelatin and stir until gelatin is completely dissolved. Remove from heat. Add egg yolks, one at a time, beating after every addition. Place pan back over boiling water; cook and stir for 2 more minutes. Remove from heat. Add vanilla extract and stir to mix thoroughly. Cool. Beat egg whites until stiff. Fold into cooled chocolate mixture. Chill until mixture starts to thicken. Fold in prepared nondairy whipped topping. Line bottom and sides of large, decorative mould with thin slices of sponge cake. Alternate layers of chocolate mixture and sponge cake to complete the torte. Chill at least 14 hours.

Yield: 20 servings
Exchange, 1 serving: ⅓ fat
Calories, 1 serving: 40

Sponge Cake

4	eggs, separated	4
3 T.	granulated sugar replacement	45 mL
½ c.	hot water	125 mL
1½ t.	vanilla extract	7 mL
1½ c.	cake flour, sifted	375 mL
¼ t.	salt	1 mL
¼ t.	baking powder	1 mL

With electric beater, beat egg yolks and sugar replacement until thick and lemon-colored. Beat in hot water and vanilla. Combine cake flour, salt and baking powder in sifter; sift and stir into the egg yolk mixture. Beat egg whites until stiff and fold into egg yolk mixture. Spoon batter into ungreased 9-in. (23-cm) tube pan. Bake at 325 °F (165 °C) for 55 to 60 minutes, or until cake is done. Invert pan and allow cake to cool at least 1 hour. Remove from pan.

Yield: 16 servings
Exchange, 1 serving: ½ bread
Calories, 1 serving: 54

Chocolate Heaven

½	Sponge Cake	½
3 oz.	baking chocolate	90 g
½ c.	skim milk	125 mL
¼ c.	granulated sugar replacement	60 mL
4	eggs, separated	4
2 t.	brandy flavoring	10 mL
dash	salt	dash
1 env.	nondairy whipped topping	1 env.

Line loaf pan with waxed paper. Cover bottom and sides with thin slices of sponge cake (save enough slices to cover top). Melt baking chocolate in top of double boiler; add skim milk and continue cooking and stirring until smooth and well blended. Slightly beat the egg yolks; add sugar replacement and a small amount of chocolate mixture. Stir to thoroughly mix and add to chocolate mixture in the double boiler. Cook until thick and smooth, stirring constantly. Remove from heat; while still hot, fold in stiffly beaten egg whites, brandy flavoring and salt. Cool slightly. Pour chocolate mixture into loaf pan lined with sponge cake. Cover with a layer of the remaining cake slices. Chill for at least 14 hours. Turn out onto a serving plate. Frost with nondairy topping.

Yield: 12 servings
Exchange, 1 serving: ⅓ bread
*   ½ medium meat*
*   ½ fat*
Calories, 1 serving: 91

Viennese Ruffles au Chocolat

Absolutely great—and look at the exchange and calorie counts.

⅔ c.	*flour, sifted*	*165 mL*
2 T.	*cocoa*	*30 mL*
½ t.	*salt*	*2 mL*
3 T.	*granulated sugar replacement*	*45 mL*
⅓ c.	*white wine*	*90 mL*
6	*egg whites, stiffly beaten*	*6*
	Powdered Sugar Replacement	

Combine flour, cocoa, salt and sugar in large mixing bowl; beat in white wine to make a medium batter. Fold stiffly beaten egg whites into mixture. Pour batter into a pastry bag with a large, plain or fluted, tube. Squeeze batter into hot, deep fat (365 °F or 180 °C) and fry until delicately browned. Drain on absorbent paper, such as paper toweling. Sprinkle lightly with powdered sugar replacement.

Yield: 30 ruffles
Exchange, 1 ruffle: ⅓ bread
Calories, 1 ruffle: 15

Pastry Cups

These will be useful in many desserts.

1	*egg*	*1*
dash	*salt*	*dash*
½ c.	*skim milk*	*125 mL*
1 t.	*vanilla extract*	*5 mL*
½ c.	*flour*	*125 mL*
	oil for deep-fat frying	

Combine egg and salt in mixing bowl; beat to blend thoroughly. Add milk, vanilla and flour, beating just to blend until smooth. Heat rosette iron in hot deep fat (365 °F or 180 °C), and shake off excess oil. Dip into batter to within ¼-in. (6-mm) of top of iron. Return to hot oil; cover iron completely with oil. Fry until golden brown. Drain on absorbent paper.

Yield: 10 pastry cups
Exchange, 1 pastry cup: ⅓ bread
Calories, 1 pastry cup: 34

Bridal Tortes

An impressive dessert for bridal showers.

1/3 c.	margarine	90 mL
1/4 c.	granulated sugar replacement	60 mL
1 oz.	baking chocolate, melted and cooled	30 g
2 t.	vanilla extract	10 mL
2	eggs	2
8	Meringue Nests	8
8 T.	nondairy whipped topping	120 mL

Cream margarine and sugar replacement until light and fluffy. Blend in baking chocolate and vanilla. Add eggs, one at a time, beating for 5 minutes after each addition. Turn into meringue nests. Chill at least 1 to 2 hours before serving. Top each shell with 1 T. (15 mL) of nondairy whipped topping.

Yield: 8 servings
Exchange, 1 serving: ½ lean meat
2 fat
Calories, 1 serving: 110

Individual Meringue Nests

Use these with almost anything—fruits, puddings, custards or ice cream.

4	egg whites	4
dash	salt	dash
1/4 t.	cream of tartar	1 mL
1/2 c.	granulated sugar replacement	125 mL
1 T.	white vinegar	15 mL
1 T.	white vanilla extract	15 mL

Beat egg whites, salt and cream of tartar into soft peaks. Gradually add granulated sugar replacement, vinegar and vanilla. Beat until mixture forms stiff peaks. Cover cookie sheet with parchment or plain paper. Draw eight 4-in. (10-cm) circles; divide meringue evenly among circles. Using the back of a spoon, shape into nests. Bake at 250 °F (120 °C) for 45 to 50 minutes. Turn off heat an allow to dry in oven for about 1 hour.

Yield: 8 servings
Exchange, 1 serving: negligible
Calories, 1 serving: negligible

Prize Chocolate Cheesecake

Crust

32	graham crackers, crumbed	32
¼ c.	margarine, melted	60 mL
2 t.	granulated sugar replacement	10 mL
½ c.	semisweet chocolate chips	125 mL

Filling

8-oz. pkg.	cream cheese	226-g pkg.
2 T.	lemon juice	30 mL
1	egg, separated	1
2 T.	granulated sugar replacement	30 mL
⅔ c.	skim milk	180 mL
½ t.	lemon rind, freshly grated	2 mL
1 env.	unflavored gelatin	1 env.
2 T.	boiling water	30 mL

Decorative Topping

¼ c.	semisweet chocolate chips, chopped	60 mL

To make the crust, mix graham cracker crumbs, margarine and sugar replacement together. Press into bottom and sides of a 9-in. (23-cm) springform pan. Chill until firm. Melt chocolate chips and spread on top of crust. Refrigerate.

For the filling, beat cream cheese with lemon juice until smooth. Place egg yolk, sugar replacement and milk in saucepan. Heat gently until thick enough to coat the back of a spoon, but DO NOT BOIL. Remove from heat. Gradually stir in the cream cheese mixture and grated lemon rind. Dissolve gelatin in boiling water. Stir into mixture and blend thoroughly. Beat egg white until stiff and fold into the filling. Pour the filling over chocolate-layered crust. Refrigerate to completely set. Decorate top with chopped chocolate chips. Refrigerate until serving time.

Yield: 20 servings
Exchange, 1 serving: 1 bread
2 fat
Calories, 1 serving: 149

Pastry with Chocolate Cheese Filling

Cake

1¾ c.	flour	440 mL
1 pkg.	dry yeast	1 pkg.
⅓ c.	sour cream	90 mL
¼ c.	margarine	60 mL
2 T.	water	30 mL
3 T.	granulated sugar replacement	45 mL
dash	salt	dash
1	egg	1

Filling

3-oz. pkg.	cream cheese	110-g pkg.
2 T.	granulated sugar replacement	30 mL
1	egg yolk	1
1 T.	sour cream	15 mL
1 oz.	baking chocolate, melted	30 g
1 T.	vanilla extract	5 mL

Topping

1	egg white, beaten	1
1 t.	granulated sugar replacement	5 mL

Sift flour and mix with the dry yeast in a large bowl. In a saucepan, blend together the sour cream, margarine, water, sugar replacement, salt and egg. Heat until warm, stirring constantly. Stir in the flour and mix into a soft dough. Knead the dough on a lightly floured surface. Place in a greased bowl and allow to rise until doubled in size.

Combine the filling ingredients and beat until thoroughly blended. Turn dough out onto lightly floured surface and knead a few times. Roll dough out into a 9 × 16-in. (23 × 40-cm) rectangle. Spread the cheese filling evenly over the dough and roll up from the longer edge to make a 16-in. (40-cm) roll. Place, seam side down, on greased cookie sheet. Set in a warm place for 45 minutes or until dough has doubled in size. Brush with topping of beaten egg white mixed with sugar replacement. Bake at 325 °F (165 °C) for 25 to 30 minutes or until golden brown. Remove from oven and serve warm.

Yield: 15 servings
Exchange, 1 serving: ¾ bread
¾ fat
Calories, 1 serving: 130

Chocolate Almond Tart

An extravagance!

Crust

¾ c.	flour, sifted	190 mL
2 t.	granulated sugar replacement	10 mL
5 T.	margarine	75 mL
½ t.	vanilla extract	2 mL
2–3 T.	water	30–45 mL

Filling

1	egg	1
1 T.	flour	15 mL
¼ c.	skim milk	60 mL
¼ c.	heavy cream	60 mL
⅓ c.	granulated sugar replacement	90 mL
1 oz.	baking chocolate, melted	30 g
½ c.	almonds, slivered	125 mL
2 t.	brandy flavoring	10 mL
dash	salt	dash

In a bowl or food processor, combine flour, sugar replacement and margarine. With a steel blade or knife work into a mixture like cornmeal. Add vanilla extract and enough water to make a soft dough. Press dough evenly into a 9-in. (23-cm) false-bottom tart pan. Chill in refrigerator for 45 minutes. Cover the chilled dough with aluminum foil and fill with dried beans or pie weights. Bake in the lower part of a 400 °F (200 °C) oven for 8 minutes. Remove foil and beans and bake the crust for 5 minutes longer. Remove from oven. Combine filling ingredients and beat well. Pour into partially baked shell. Set on the middle rack of the oven and bake for 20 to 30 minutes, until filling is set and a knife inserted in center comes out clean. Cool.

Yield: 14 servings
Exchange, 1 serving: ½ bread
2 fat
Calories, 1 serving: 120

Butterscotch-Chocolate Charlotte Russe

1 env.	unflavored gelatin	1 env.
¼ c.	cold water	60 mL
1 c.	skim evaporated milk	250 mL
1 T.	butter	15 mL
1 oz.	baking chocolate	30 g
⅓ c.	granulated brown sugar replacement	60 mL
1½ c.	skim milk	375 mL
2	eggs, separated	2
dash	salt	dash
¼ t.	vanilla extract	1 mL
12	ladyfingers	12

Soften gelatin in cold water; set aside. Pour skim evaporated milk into freezer tray and place in freezer to thoroughly chill until edges are slightly frozen. Melt butter and baking chocolate in top of double boiler. Add brown sugar replacement and cook until well blended. Add milk. Heat and stir until warm. Pour over well-beaten egg yolks, stirring constantly. Add salt and return to top of double boiler. Cook over hot water, stirring constantly, until mixture coats a spoon. Remove from heat and add softened gelatin. Stir until dissolved. Chill until mixture begins to thicken. Beat egg whites until stiff and fold into the cooled chocolate mixture. In chilled mixing bowl, combine vanilla extract and slightly frozen evaporated milk and beat until stiff. Fold into mixture. Pour into a decorative mould lined with separated ladyfingers. Chill until firm. Unmould onto a serving plate.

Yield: 8 servings
Exchange, 1 serving: 1 low-fat milk
⅔ fat
Calories, 1 serving: 112

Schaum Torte

3	egg whites	3
dash	salt	dash
dash	cream of tartar	dash mL
2 T.	granulated sugar replacement	30 mL
2 t.	white vinegar	10 mL
1 t.	white vanilla extract	5 mL
2 oz.	dietetic white chocolate	60 g
10	fresh strawberries, whole	10

Beat egg whites with salt until frothy; add cream of tartar and beat until whites stand in soft peaks. Gradually, add sugar replacement; continue beating and add vinegar and white vanilla extract. Lightly grease bottom of 9-in. (23-cm) springform pan. Spread mixture into pan. Bake at 250 °F (120 °C) for 50 to 60 minutes. Remove from oven and release side of pan. Cool completely. Melt dietetic white chocolate in top of double boiler; gently pour to drizzle over top of torte. Cool. Decorate with fresh strawberries.

Yield: 10 servings
Exchange, 1 serving: ⅓ bread
⅓ fat
Calories, 1 serving: 31

Chocolate Blitz Torte

My first choice among tortes.

1 c.	cake flour, sifted	250 mL
1 t.	baking powder	5 mL
dash	salt	dash
⅓ c.	vegetable shortening, softened	90 mL
2 oz.	baking chocolate, melted	60 g
⅔ c.	granulated sugar replacement	180 mL
4	eggs, separated	4
1 t.	vanilla extract	5 mL
3 T.	skim milk	45 mL
2 t.	sorbitol	10 mL
½ c.	almonds, slivered	125 mL
½ recipe	Chocolate Whipped Topping	½ recipe

Sift cake flour, baking powder and salt together. Cream shortening, melted chocolate and sugar replacement until light and fluffy. Add well-beaten egg yolks, vanilla extract and skim milk. Beat until thoroughly blended. Beat in flour mixture. Divide batter and spread into 2 well-greased 9-in. (23-cm) baking pans. Beat egg whites until stiff; add sorbitol and continue beating to completely mix. Divide and spread over batter in both baking pans. Sprinkle with slivered almonds. Bake at 350 °F (175 °C) for 25 to 30 minutes. Cool; spread chocolate whipped topping between the layers.

Yield: 20 servings
Exchange, 1 serving: ⅓ bread
1 fat
Calories, 1 serving: 81

Chocolate Charlotte Russe

1 env.	unflavored gelatin	1 env.
3 T.	cold water	45 mL
1 oz.	baking chocolate	30 g
¼ c.	boiling water	60 mL
¼ c.	granulated sugar replacement	60 mL
dash	salt	dash
1¾ c.	skim evaporated milk	440 mL
1 t.	vanilla extract	5 mL
10	ladyfingers	10

Soften gelatin in cold water for 5 minutes. Melt baking chocolate in top of double boiler; add boiling water and cook slowly, stirring constantly, to a smooth and thick paste. Add sugar replacement, salt and ¾ c. (190 mL) of the evaporated milk. Cook and stir 5 minutes longer. Remove from heat and add softened gelatin, stirring until gelatin is dissolved. Cool. Place remaining evaporated milk in a freezer tray and freeze until thoroughly chilled and edges are slightly frozen. When chocolate mixture begins to thicken and cool, whip slightly frozen milk until stiff and fold into cooled chocolate mixture with the vanilla. Line a decorative mould with the ladyfingers and pour the chocolate mixture into the mould. Chill until firm; unmould onto a serving plate.

Yield: 8 servings
Exchange, 1 serving: ⅔ bread
½ fat
Calories, 1 serving: 81

Chocolate Rum Torte

¼ c.	boiling water	60 mL
¼ c.	chocolate chips	60 mL
4	eggs, separated	4
3 t.	rum flavoring	15 mL
32	vanilla wafers	32
⅓ c.	water	90 mL

In a saucepan, pour boiling water over chocolate chips and stir to melt chips. Beat egg yolks, one at a time, into the chocolate mixture. Place pan over low heat and cook until thick. Remove from heat and cool completely. Add 1 t. (5 mL) of the rum flavoring. Beat egg whites until stiff. Fold small amount of whites into chocolate mixture to lighten, then fold chocolate mixture into remaining egg whites. In a small cup, dilute the remaining 2 t. (10 mL) rum flavoring with ⅓ c. (90 mL) water. Dip each wafer into flavoring. Place the 16 dipped wafers on bottom of 8-in. (20-cm) springform pan, spread with half of chocolate mixture, top with remaining 16 dipped wafers, spread remaining chocolate mixture over top. Freeze until firm.

Yield: 20 servings
Exchange, 1 serving: ½ bread
½ fat
Calories, 1 serving: 55

Quick Pastries

Quick Pastry Dessert

1 recipe	Pastry Cups	1 recipe
1 pkg.	low-cal chocolate pudding mix	1 pkg.
2 c.	skim milk	500 mL
1 t.	unflavored gelatin	5 mL
1 t.	cinnamon	5 mL
1	egg white	1
1 c.	nondairy whipped topping	250 mL

Prepare pastry cups as directed in recipe. Cool completely. Combine pudding mix and milk in saucepan; add gelatin and cinnamon. Cook and stir as directed on package until pudding is very thick. Cool. Beat egg white until very stiff. Fold into pudding mixture. Refrigerate until completely set. Fill pastry cups. Turn nondairy whipped topping into decorative pastry tube. Decorate tops of pastries.

Yield: 10 servings
Exchange, 1 serving: ¾ bread
Calories, 1 serving: 67

Quick Chocolate Cheesecake

Crust and Topping

¼ c.	margarine	60 mL
32	graham crackers, crumbed	32

Filling

1¼ c.	skim milk	310 mL
1 pkg.	low-cal chocolate pudding mix	1 pkg.
1 c.	cottage cheese (low-cal)	250 mL
1 c.	nondairy whipped topping	250 mL

Melt the margarine and mix with graham cracker crumbs; reserve ¼ c. (60 mL) for the topping. Press remaining crumbs into the base of an 8-in. (20-cm) flan ring set on a serving plate. Refrigerate to firm.

For the filling, combine skim milk and chocolate pudding mix in saucepan. Cook and stir over medium heat until mixture is thick. Remove from heat. Turn cottage cheese into blender or food processor and blend to thoroughly cream. Stir into the pudding. Cool slightly. Fold nondairy whipped topping into pudding. Spoon mixture over crumb crust. Chill until firm. Remove the flan ring and decorate with reserved graham cracker crumbs.

Yield: 8 servings
Exchange, 1 serving: 2 bread
½ high-fat meat
1 fat
Calories, 1 serving: 237

Delectable Crèmes

Great Lakes Pudding

Inspired by the region where I was born.

Pudding

3 c.	wide noodles, uncooked	750 mL
2	eggs, beaten	2
½ c.	cottage cheese (low-cal)	125 mL
⅓ c.	sour cream	90 mL
¼ c.	granulated sugar replacement	60 mL
¾ c.	skim milk	190 mL
1 oz.	baking chocolate, melted	30 g
1 T.	margarine	15 mL
1 t.	vanilla extract	5 mL

Topping

½ c.	unsweetened cornflakes	125 mL
1 T.	margarine, melted	15 mL
1 t.	granulated sugar replacement	5 mL

Cook noodles in boiling water until tender. Drain, rinse and cool thoroughly. Set aside. In large bowl, combine eggs, cottage cheese, sour cream and sugar replacement and stir until smooth. Add skim milk, melted chocolate, margarine and vanilla extract. Mix thoroughly. Stir in noodles and blend well. Cover and refrigerate overnight. Pour noodle mixture into a greased 8-in. (20-cm) baking dish. Combine topping ingredients in mixing bowl and lightly stir to blend. Sprinkle evenly over pudding. Bake at 350 °F (175 °C) for 40 to 50 minutes until topping is golden brown. Serve warm.

Yield: 9 servings
Exchange, 1 serving: 1 bread
1 high-fat meat
Calories, 1 serving: 164

Pouding de Riz

Adapted from a Haitian rice pudding.

4	egg yolks	4
3 T.	granulated sugar replacement	45 mL
dash	salt	dash
1½ t.	vanilla extract	7 mL
1 qt.	skim milk, hot	1 L
1½ c.	cooked rice	375 mL
½ c.	semisweet chocolate chips	125 mL
4	egg whites	4
3 pkg.	aspartame sweetener	3 pkg.

In a mixing bowl, beat egg yolks with the sugar replacement and salt until pale yellow in color and slightly thickened. Stir in 1 teaspoon (5 mL) of the vanilla. Stir egg yolk mixture into the hot milk and cook, stirring, until custard coats the spoon. BE CAREFUL NOT TO LET MIXTURE BOIL. Add rice and chocolate chips; stir to completely mix. Pour into greased 1-qt. (1-L) baking dish. Bake at 350 °F (175 °C) for 10 minutes. Meanwhile, beat egg whites until stiff but not dry. Beat in aspartame sweetener. Stir in the remaining vanilla extract. Remove pudding from oven, spread the egg white mixture over the pudding. Place pudding back in oven, bake for 5 minutes more or until meringue is slightly brown.

Yield: 8 servings
Exchange, 1 serving: 1 medium-fat milk
                    1 fruit
Calories, 1 serving: 176

Regal Custard

5 T.	granulated sugar replacement	70 mL
3 c.	skim milk, hot	750 mL
8	egg yolks	8
1½ t.	vanilla extract	7 mL
3 T.	crème de cacao	45 mL
6	egg whites	6

Add 2 T. (30 mL) of the sugar replacement to skim milk and stir to dissolve. Beat egg yolks until frothy; gradually beat in hot milk mixture. Add vanilla extract. Pour into a well-greased 2-qt. (2-L) baking dish. Bake at 350 °F (175 °C) for 35 to 45 minutes or until a knife comes out clean. Remove from oven. Pour crème de cacao over the surface. Beat egg whites until stiff and gradually beat in the remaining 3 T. (45 mL) of the sugar replacement and vanilla extract. Spread half the meringue over the custard. Decorate with remaining meringue by pressing it through a pastry tube or dropping it from a teaspoon. Return to oven and bake for 12 to 15 minutes or until meringue is a delicate brown.

Yield: 12 servings
Exchange, 1 serving: ⅓ bread
½ high-fat meat
Calories, 1 serving: 74

Chocolate Pear Whip

4	pears	4
1 T.	lemon juice	15 mL
dash	salt	dash
3	egg whites	3
2 T.	granulated sugar replacement	30 mL
1 oz.	baking chocolate, melted	30 g

Peel, core and cube pears; place in blender. Blend into a soft purée. Mix purée, lemon juice and salt together. Beat egg whites until soft peaks form. Gradually, add sugar replacement and pear purée. Fold in chocolate to marbleize.

Yield: 8 servings
Exchange, 1 serving: 1 bread
½ fat
Calories, 1 serving: 89

Cocoa Cream Tapioca

2⅔ c.	skim milk	680 mL
3 T.	granulated sugar replacement	45 mL
¼ t.	salt	1 mL
¼ c.	cocoa	60 mL
¼ c.	quick-cooking tapioca	60 mL
½ t.	vanilla extract	2 mL
2 t.	butter	10 mL

In top of double boiler, bring skim milk to boiling point; stir in sugar replacement, salt, cocoa and tapioca. Cook over boiling water until translucent and soft. Add vanilla extract and butter. Pour into serving dishes. Press waxed paper directly onto surface of pudding. Chill. Remove paper just before serving.

Yield: 10 servings
Exchange, 1 serving: ½ bread
Calories, 1 serving: 42

Cocoa Rice Pudding

1½ c.	cooked rice	375 mL
¼ c.	cocoa	60 mL
3 T.	granulated sugar replacement	45 mL
1 t.	vanilla extract	5 mL
2	eggs, separated	2
⅛ t.	salt	½ mL
¼ t.	cream of tartar	1 mL

Combine cooked rice, cocoa, sugar replacement, vanilla and egg yolks in mixing bowl. Stir to blend completely. Beat egg whites with salt and cream of tartar into stiff peaks. Gently fold egg whites into cocoa mixture. Pour into a greased 1-qt. (1-L) baking dish. Bake at 350 °F (175 °C) for 15 to 20 minutes or until pudding is set.

Yield: 8 servings
Exchange, 1 serving: ⅔ bread
½ fat
Calories, 1 serving: 67

Chocolate Custard with "Snow" Mounds

2 c.	skim milk	500 mL
1/4 c.	skim evaporated milk	60 mL
2 T.	granulated sugar replacement	30 mL
1/2	vanilla bean, split	1/2
4	eggs, separated	4
2 T.	sorbitol	30 mL
1 oz.	baking chocolate, melted	30 g

In a large saucepan, combine skim milk, evaporated milk, sugar replacement and vanilla bean. Bring to a simmer. Beat egg whites until stiff and gradually beat in the sorbitol to make a smooth meringue. Drop meringue by tablespoons into the simmering milk mixture, turning each mound over two or three times as it poaches. Poach for about 3 minutes. (**Do not overcrowd pan when poaching**.) Remove meringues and drain on a towel. Stir melted chocolate into custard mixture. Beat egg yolks and gradually pour hot milk mixture over them. Stir continuously. Pour mixture back into saucepan. Return saucepan to low heat on stove. Stir until custard thickens. Pour custard into 6 individual serving dishes. Top with meringue mounds.

Yield: 8 servings
Exchange, 1 serving: ½ high-fat meat
⅓ no-fat milk
Calories, 1 serving: 86

Aladdin's Crème

Smooth and creamy, a treat for the whole family.

1	egg	1
1/3 c.	granulated sugar replacement	90 mL
2 oz.	baking chocolate, melted	60 g
1/2 c.	skim milk	125 mL
2 t.	unsalted butter, melted	10 mL
1 c.	all-purpose flour	250 mL
1 T.	baking powder	15 mL
1/4 t.	salt	1 mL
1 t.	vanilla extract	5 mL

Beat egg and granulated sugar replacement until well blended and frothy. Add baking chocolate, milk, butter, flour, baking powder, salt and vanilla extract. Beat until thoroughly blended and smooth. Pour into a well-greased 1½-qt. (1½-L) mould or baking dish. Place a rack in a large saucepan on top of the stove. Add boiling water to level of the rack. Place mould with pudding on rack. Cover saucepan and keep water boiling over low heat to steam the crème. Cook for 1½ hours or until crème is set.

Yield: 14 servings
Exchange, 1 serving: ½ bread
¾ fat
Calories, 1 serving: 68

French Crème

The little extra work is well worth the trouble.

3 T.	granulated sugar replacement	45 mL
3 T.	cocoa	45 mL
2 T.	all-purpose flour	30 mL
3	egg yolks	3
1	egg	1
dash	salt	dash
1 c.	skim milk, hot	250 mL
1 t.	vanilla extract	5 mL
1 T.	margarine	15 mL
1 T.	almond paste	15 mL
1 T.	coconut, finely grated	15 mL

In the top of a double boiler combine sugar replacement, cocoa, flour, egg yolks, egg and salt. Stir in skim milk. Cook and stir over simmering water until crème is smooth and thick. Remove from heat and stir in vanilla extract, margarine, almond paste and coconut. Pour into 4 individual serving dishes. Serve hot.

Yield: 4 servings
Exchange, 1 serving: ¾ high-fat milk
⅓ fat
Calories, 1 serving: 140

Creamy Chocolate Mousse

An American favorite.

⅓ c.	cocoa	90 mL
1 t.	instant coffee	5 mL
¼ c.	granulated sugar replacement	60 mL
2 T.	cornstarch	30 mL
¼ t.	salt	1 mL
2 c.	skim milk	500 mL
1	egg, beaten	1
8 oz.	cream cheese, softened	240 g
1 t.	vanilla extract	5 mL

Combine cocoa, coffee, sugar replacement, cornstarch and salt in saucepan; stir in milk. Cook and stir over medium heat until thick and bubbly; reduce heat, and then cook and stir 4 minutes more. Remove from heat. Stir small amount of hot mixture into beaten egg and pour egg mixture into hot mixture, stirring to blend. Cook over low heat for 2 minutes and remove from heat. Add cream cheese and vanilla, beating until well blended and fluffy. Pour into 1-qt. (1-L) mould or dish. Cover with waxed paper and chill until firm. Remove paper and unmould.

Yield: 10 servings
Exchange, 1 serving: 1 full-fat milk
1 fat
Calories, 1 serving: 128

Fructose Custard

The vanilla bean gives it that special flavor.

2 c.	skim milk	500 mL
3 T.	liquid fructose	45 mL
3 T.	cocoa	45 mL
1	vanilla bean, split	1
4	egg yolks	4

Combine milk, liquid fructose and cocoa in saucepan. Stir to completely mix. Add vanilla bean. Heat to the scalding point, stirring often; remove from heat. In a separate bowl, beat egg yolks until thick. Remove vanilla bean from the chocolate/milk mixture. Very gradually beat the hot milk into the egg yolks. Pour the mixture into the saucepan. Continue cooking and stirring over very low heat until the custard thickens. Pour into 4 individual custard cups. Chill.

Yield: 4 servings
Exchange, 1 serving: ½ bread
               1 medium-fat meat
Calories, 1 serving: 115

Chocolate Banana Mousse

1 oz.	unsweetened chocolate	30 g
1 c.	skim evaporated milk	250 mL
3 T.	granulated sugar replacement	45 mL
2	egg yolks	2
¼ t.	salt	1 mL
1 t.	vanilla extract	5 mL
2	bananas, sliced	2

Combine chocolate, ¼ c. (60 mL) of the milk and the sugar replacement in top of double boiler. (Chill remaining milk in freezer.) Cook and stir over simmering water until chocolate melts. Pour small amount of hot chocolate mixture over egg yolks and beat well. Pour egg mixture into chocolate mixture in top of double boiler. Stir in salt. Cook and stir over hot water until mixture thickens. Cool completely. Scrape cold or slightly frozen milk into mixing bowl and beat until very stiff. Fold chocolate mixture into stiffly beaten milk. Fold in vanilla and banana slices. Spoon into mould, freezer tray or individual cups and freeze until firm.

Yield: 8 servings
Exchange, 1 serving: 1 bread
               ½ fat
Calories, 1 serving: 69

Chocolate Cream-of-Rice

A rice pudding like you have never tasted before.

½ c.	rice flour	125 mL
3 T.	granulated sugar replacement	45 mL
½ c.	skim milk	125 mL
4	eggs	4
1 oz.	baking chocolate	30 g
2 T.	water	30 mL
3	egg whites, beaten stiff	3
1	grated rind of 1 orange	1

Mix rice flour, sugar replacement and milk in mixing bowl. Beat in eggs. Combine baking chocolate and water in small saucepan; stir over low heat to melt chocolate. Fold melted chocolate, egg whites and orange rind into rice flour mixture. Pour into a greased and sugared (use sugar replacement) charlotte mould. Bake at 350 °F (175 °C) for 20 to 25 minutes or until crème tests done.

Yield: 6 servings
Exchange, 1 serving: 1 medium-fat milk
Calories, 1 serving: 121

Marshmallow Crème and Marshmallows

3 env.	unflavored gelatin	3 env.
¼ c.	cold water	60 mL
¾ c.	boiling water	190 mL
3 T.	granulated sugar replacement or granulated fructose	45 mL
1 t.	white vanilla extract	5 mL
3	egg whites	3

Sprinkle gelatin over cold water in mixing bowl; set aside 5 minutes to soften. Add to boiling water in a saucepan; cook and stir until gelatin is dissolved. Remove from heat. Cool to consistency of thick syrup. Add sugar replacement and vanilla, stirring to blend. Beat egg whites into soft peaks. Very slowly, trickle a small stream of gelatin mixture into egg whites, beating until all gelatin mixture is blended. Continue beating until light and fluffy. Pour into prepared pan.

To form the marshmallows: Fill 13 × 9 × 2-in. (33 × 23 × 5-cm) pan with flour or cornstarch to desired depth. Form moulds using a small glass, the inside of a dough cutter or any object of desired size by pressing the form into flour to the bottom of the pan. Spoon marshmallow crème into the moulds and refrigerate until set. Dust or roll tops in flour; shake off excess. Store in refrigerator.

Yield: 4 c. (1 mL)
Exchange, 1 c. (250 mL): negligible
Calories, 1 c. (250 mL): 11

Chocolate Marshmallow Pudding

⅓ c.	cocoa	90 mL
3 c.	skim milk	750 mL
⅓ c.	granulated sugar replacement	90 mL
dash	salt	dash
3 T.	flour	45 mL
1	egg, well beaten	1
3 T.	water	45 mL
1 t.	vanilla extract	5 mL
12	Marshmallows	12

Combine the cocoa and the milk in a saucepan. Stir to blend and scald. Mix together the sugar replacement, salt, flour, egg and water to make a paste. Pour about half of the scalded milk mixture over the egg mixture, stir to blend. Return to saucepan and cook until mixture just begins to boil. Remove from heat and add vanilla extract. Pour into a well-greased 1½-qt. (1½-L) baking dish or casserole. Top with marshmallows and bake until delicate brown in a hot oven of 400 °F (200 °C). Chill and serve cold.

Yield: 12 servings
Exchange, 1 serving: ⅗ bread
Calories, 1 serving: 42

C & C Tureen

Chestnuts and chocolate—an unbeatable combination.

1 lb.	chestnuts	500 g
1/3 c.	sweet butter	90 mL
2 oz.	German chocolate, grated	60 g
2 T.	granulated sugar replacement	30 mL
1 t.	vanilla extract	5 mL

With a sharp knife slit shells of the chestnuts on convex side. Put chestnuts in a saucepan with enough water to cover, bring to a boil and simmer for 5 minutes. Remove pan from heat and remove chestnuts, one by one. Remove shells and inner skins while the nuts are still hot. Return peeled nuts to boiling water and cook for 20 minutes or until tender. Drain and place nuts in blender; blend into a purée.

Combine chestnut purée, butter, chocolate, sugar replacement and vanilla extract in bowl and stir to completely mix. Press mixture firmly into a greased paper-lined loaf pan. Chill 6 to 8 hours or overnight. Unmould the loaf onto a serving plate; cut into thin slices. Serve on chilled plates.

Yield: 8 servings
Exchange, 1 serving: ¾ bread
3 fat
Calories, 1 serving: 182

Chocolate Bread Pudding

Ol'-fashioned—but now with chocolate!

½ c.	chocolate chips	125 mL
3 c.	skim milk	750 mL
2	eggs	2
½ t.	salt	2 mL
1/3 c.	granulated sugar replacement	90 mL
2 t.	vanilla extract	10 mL
8 slices	dry bread	8 slices

Melt the chocolate chips in 1 c. (250 mL) of the skim milk over medium heat. Stir in the remaining milk. Set aside. Beat eggs until frothy; add salt, sugar replacement and vanilla extract. Beat well. Stir egg mixture into chocolate/milk mixture. Trim crusts from bread and cut slices into small cubes. Drop cubes into greased 1½-qt. (1½-L) casserole or baking dish. Pour chocolate mixture over the bread cubes; be sure to saturate all the cubes. Set casserole in pan of hot water. Bake at 350 °F (175 °C) for 1 hour or until pudding is completely set. Serve warm or cold.

Yield: 14 servings
Exchange, 1 serving: 1 bread
½ fat
Calories, 1 serving: 99

Pioneer Cornstarch Crème

2 oz.	*baking chocolate*	*60 g*
3 c.	*skim milk*	*750 mL*
½ c.	*granulated sugar replacement*	*125 mL*
¼ c.	*cornstarch*	*60 mL*
¼ t.	*salt*	*1 mL*
¼ c.	*water*	*60 mL*
2 t.	*vanilla extract*	*10 mL*
1 T.	*margarine*	*15 mL*

Melt baking chocolate in top of double boiler over simmering water; add skim milk. Stir until well blended. In shaker bottle or bowl combine the sugar replacement, cornstarch and salt with water. Shake or stir to blend well. Add to chocolate/milk mixture in double boiler. Cook and stir until thickened. Cook 20 minutes longer. Remove from heat, add vanilla extract and margarine. Spoon into serving dishes and press waxed paper directly to crème surface. Chill. Remove paper before serving.

Yield: 8 servings
Exchange, 1 serving: ¾ bread
1 fat
Calories, 1 serving: 103

New England Baked Chocolate Custard

3	eggs	3
3 T.	dietetic maple syrup	45 mL
2 c.	skim milk	500 mL
1 oz.	baking chocolate, melted	30 g
1 t.	vanilla extract	5 mL

Beat eggs until foamy and light. Add dietetic maple syrup, skim milk, melted chocolate and vanilla extract; beat until thoroughly mixed. Pour the custard mixture into 4 individual custard cups. Set the cups in a pan of hot water which comes halfway up the sides of the custard cups. Bake at 350 °F (175 °C) for 35 to 40 minutes or until knife inserted in center of custard comes out clean. Serve hot or cold.

Yield: 4 servings
Exchange, 1 serving: 1 bread
1 high-fat meat
Calories, 1 serving: 166

American Snow Cream

My children love it.

½ c.	skim milk	125 mL
1 T.	granulated sugar replacement	15 mL
1 pkg.	nondairy topping mix	1 pkg.
1 oz.	baking chocolate, melted	30 g
½ t.	vanilla extract	2 mL
2 qt.	fresh snow	2 L

Stir skim milk, sugar replacement, topping mix, baking chocolate and vanilla extract until well blended. Place fresh snow in large metal bowl. Place bowl with snow into another larger bowl which has been filled with ice. On high speed, beat chocolate mixture into snow until thick and well blended. Serve at once.

Yield: 8 servings
Exchange, 1 serving: ⅓ bread
½ fat
Calories, 1 serving: 44

Palate-Pleasing Pies

Chocolate Cream Pie

2½ c.	skim milk	625 mL
2 oz.	baking chocolate	60 g
2 T.	flour	30 mL
3 T.	cornstarch	45 L
¼ c.	granulated sugar replacement	60 mL
½ t.	salt	2 mL
4	egg yolks, beaten	4
1 T.	butter	15 mL
1½ t.	vanilla extract	7 mL
10 in.	Basic Pie Shell, baked	25 cm
1 c.	low-cal whipped topping	250 mL

Combine 2. (500 mL) of the milk with baking chocolate in top of double boiler. Cook and stir over simmering water until chocolate has melted and mixture is smooth. Sift together twice the flour, cornstarch, sugar replacement and salt. Mix flour mixture with remaining ½ c. (125 mL) milk. Add to chocolate mixture, stirring constantly, until thickened. Cook 10 minutes longer. Remove from heat, gradually add some of the chocolate mixture to the beaten egg yolks, then stir into the pan and return to heat. Cook 2 minutes longer; remove from heat, add butter and vanilla. Pour into baked pie shell. Chill in refrigerator until cool and set. Decorate with whipped topping.

Yield: 8 servings
Exchange, 1 serving: ¾ bread
2 fat
plus piecrust exchange
Calories, 1 serving: 147
plus piecrust calories

Angel Pie

Crust

4	egg whites	4
¼ t.	cream of tartar	1 mL
3 T.	granulated sugar replacement	45 mL

Beat egg whites until frothy; add cream of tartar and sugar replacement. Beat until stiff. Line a 9-in. (23-cm) pie pan with meringue mixture. Bake at 275 °F (135 °C) for 45 minutes.

Filling

4	egg yolks	4
3 T.	granulated sugar replacement	45 mL
1 oz.	baking chocolate, melted	30 g
dash	salt	dash
1 c.	low-cal whipped topping	250 mL

Beat egg yolks in top of double boiler; add sugar replacement, baking chocolate and salt. Cook and stir until thick, about 10 minutes. Cool. Fold in whipped topping. Pour mixture into angel shell.

Yield: 8 servings
Exchange, 1 serving: ½ bread
                            1 fat
                            plus piecrust exchange
Calories, 1 serving: 70
                            plus piecrust calories

South Seas Pie

¼ c.	unsweetened coconut, shredded	60 mL
9 in.	Basic Pie Shell, unbaked	23 cm
1 c.	water	250 mL
2 T.	cornstarch	30 mL
⅓ c.	mini chocolate chips	90 mL
4	eggs, slightly beaten	4
2 T.	granulated sugar replacement	30 mL
¼ t.	salt	1 mL
1½ t.	vanilla extract	7 mL
1 c.	unsalted macadamia nuts, finely chopped	250 mL

Press unsweetened coconut into bottom and sides of unbaked pie shell. Set aside. Combine water and cornstarch in saucepan, cook and stir over medium heat until mixture is thick and clear. Remove from heat and stir in mini chocolate chips. Cool to room temperature. Add eggs, sugar replacement, salt and vanilla extract. Beat with electric mixer until fluffy; fold in macadamia nuts. Pour into pie shell. Bake 325 °F (165 °C) for 40 to 45 minutes or until filling is set. Cool.

Yield: 8 servings
Exchange, 1 serving: ¾ bread
3 fat
plus piecrust exchange
Calories, 1 serving: 186
plus piecrust calories

Creamy Custard Pie

2 c.	skim milk	500 mL
¼ c.	flour	60 mL
¼ c.	cocoa	60 mL
⅛ t.	salt	1 mL
3 T.	granulated sugar replacement	45 mL
3	egg yolks	3
1 T.	butter	15 mL
1 T.	vanilla extract	15 mL
8 in.	Basic Pie Shell, baked	20 cm

Scald 1 c. (250 mL) of the milk. Mix dry ingredients with remaining milk. Add to hot milk and cook until custard coats the spoon, about 15 minutes. Add butter and vanilla. Stir to blend. Remove from heat. When partially cooled, pour into baked pie shell. Chill thoroughly before serving.

Yield: 8 servings
Exchange, 1 serving: ½ bread
1 fat
plus piecrust exchange
Calories, 1 serving: 81
plus piecrust calories

Banana Chocolate Pie

⅓ c.	flour	90 mL
3 T.	granulated sugar replacement	45 mL
⅛ t.	salt	½ mL
2 c.	skim milk, scalded	500 mL
3	egg yolks, beaten	3
1 T.	butter	15 mL
1 t.	vanilla extract	5 mL
2	bananas, sliced	2
¼ c.	mini chocolate chips	60 mL
9 in.	Basic Pie Shell, baked	23 cm

Combine flour, sugar replacement and salt in top of double boiler. Blend in milk slowly. Cook until thickened. Add beaten egg yolks and cook 2 minutes longer, stirring constantly. Remove from heat, add butter and vanilla extract. Cool. Add sliced bananas and chocolate chips. Fold to completely blend. Turn into baked pie shell. Chill for at least 2 hours before serving.

Yield: 8 servings
Exchange, 1 serving: ¾ lean meat
½ fruit
plus piecrust exchange
Calories, 1 serving: 129
plus piecrust calories

Favorite Pie

1 env.	unflavored gelatin	1 env.
¼ c.	cold water	60 mL
2 oz.	baking chocolate	60 g
1 c.	skim milk	250 mL
3	egg yolks, beaten	3
3 T.	granulated sugar replacement	45 mL
¼ t.	salt	1 mL
3	egg whites	3
¼ t.	cream of tartar	1 mL
2 c.	low-cal whipped topping	500 mL
9 in.	Basic Pie Shell, baked	23 cm

Soften gelatin in water. Melt chocolate in top of double boiler; add gelatin, beaten egg yolks, sugar replacement and salt. Cook in double boiler until thick. Cool. Beat egg whites and cream of tartar until stiff; fold into chilled chocolate mixture. Fold whipped topping into chocolate mixture. Pour into baked pie shell. Chill for at least 3 hours.

Yield: 8 servings
Exchange, 1 serving: ½ full-fat milk
⅓ fat
plus piecrust exchange
Calories, 1 serving: 101
plus piecrust calories

Chocolate Rum Pie

A **must** for senior citizens' dinners.

9 in.	Basic Pie Shell, baked	23 cm
1 env.	unflavored gelatin	1 env.
1 c.	skim milk	250 mL
2	eggs, separated	2
2 T.	granulated sugar replacement	30 mL
dash	salt	dash
¼ c.	cocoa	60 mL
2 t.	rum flavoring	10 mL
1 T.	liquid sugar replacement	15 mL
2 c.	low-cal whipped topping	500 mL

Prepare and bake pie shell. Combine gelatin, milk, egg yolks, granulated sugar replacement, salt and cocoa in heavy saucepan. Cook and stir over low heat until completely blended and slightly thickened. Remove from heat. Stir in rum flavoring and chill until partially set. Beat egg whites and liquid sugar replacement into stiff peaks and fold into cooled chocolate mixture. Layer chocolate mixture and topping into baked pie shell, ending with topping. Chill until firm.

Yield: 8 servings
Exchange, 1 serving: ½ high-fat meat
⅓ fruit
plus piecrust exchange
Calories, 1 serving: 74
plus piecrust calories

Holiday Feast Pie

With all those calories—it **has** to be kept for holidays!

8 oz.	cream cheese, softened	226 g
1 c.	pumpkin purée	250 mL
¼ c.	granulated brown sugar replacement	60 mL
3	eggs, beaten	3
1½ T.	flour	25 mL
¼ t.	allspice	1 mL
⅓ c.	milk chocolate chips	90 mL
9 in.	Basic Pie Shell, baked	23 cm
2 c.	low-cal whipped topping	500 mL

Place cream cheese in top of double boiler. Using an electric mixer, beat until smooth. Add pumpkin, brown sugar replacement, eggs, flour and allspice and continue beating until completely blended and smooth. Cook and stir over simmering water until mixture thickens. Cool slightly. Fold in milk chocolate chips. Pour into baked pie shell. Chill until filling is set. Top with whipped topping.

Yield: 8 servings
Exchange, 1 serving: 1 bread
3 fat
plus piecrust exchange
Calories, 1 serving: 197
plus piecrust calories

Butterscotch Pie

¼ c.	granulated brown sugar replacement	60 mL
⅓ c.	flour	90 mL
½ t.	salt	2 mL
2½ c.	skim milk	625 mL
⅓ c.	Chocolate Syrup	90 mL
2	egg yolks, well beaten	2
1 T.	margarine	15 mL
½ t.	vanilla extract	2 mL
9 in.	Basic Pie Shell, baked	23 cm

In a saucepan, combine brown sugar replacement, flour, salt, milk, chocolate syrup and beaten egg yolks. Cook and stir over medium heat until thick. Remove from heat, blend in margarine and vanilla extract. Pour into baked pie shell. Chill in refrigerator at least 3 hours before serving or until mixture is set and cool.

Yield: 8 servings
Exchange, 1 serving: ½ bread
1 fat
plus piecrust exchange
Calories, 1 serving: 74
plus piecrust calories

Maple-Nut Chocolate Pie

A New England turnabout.

1 env.	unflavored gelatin	1 env.
2 T.	cold water	30 mL
½ c.	skim milk	125 mL
⅓ c.	low-cal maple syrup	90 mL
¼ c.	semisweet mini chocolate chips	60 mL
⅛ t.	salt	½ mL
2	egg yolks	2
1 c.	low-cal whipped topping	250 mL
2	egg whites, beaten stiff	2
¼ c.	walnuts, chopped	60 mL
9 in.	Basic Pie Shell, baked	23 cm

Soften gelatin in water. Combine milk, syrup, chocolate chips, salt and egg yolks in top of double boiler. Cook and stir until mixture is thickened. Add gelatin and stir to dissolve completely. Allow mixture to cool. Fold whipped topping into cooled mixture. Carefully fold egg whites into mixture. Fold in nuts and pour entire mixture into baked pie shell. Refrigerate until set.

Yield: 8 servings
Exchange, 1 serving: 1 bread
1 fat
plus piecrust exchanges
Calories, 1 serving: 106
plus piecrust calories

Granny's Chocolate Pie

2 T.	flour	30 mL
¼ c.	granulated sugar replacement	60 mL
3 T.	cocoa	45 mL
2 T.	butter, melted	30 mL
2	eggs	2
1 c.	buttermilk	250 mL
1 t.	vanilla extract	5 mL
9 in.	Basic Pie Shell, unbaked	23 cm

In a mixing bowl, stir flour, sugar replacement and cocoa until well blended. With an electric mixer on low speed, beat in melted butter. Beat in eggs until thoroughly blended. Beat in buttermilk and vanilla. Pour mixture into pie shell. Bake at 350 °F (175 °C) for 1 hour or until filling is set.

Yield: 8 servings
Exchange, 1 serving: ⅓ bread
1 fat
plus piecrust exchange
Calories, 1 Serving: 53
plus piecrust calories

Coconut Chocolate Pie

3 T.	cocoa	45 mL
2 T.	granulated sugar replacement	30 mL
3	eggs, well beaten	3
⅛ t.	salt	½ mL
1 t.	vanilla extract	5 mL
¼ c.	unsweetened coconut, chopped	60 mL
2 c.	skim milk, scalded	500 mL
9 in.	Basic Pie Shell, unbaked	23 cm

Blend cocoa, sugar replacement, eggs, salt, vanilla and coconut. Add scalded milk slowly. Pour into unbaked pie shell. Bake at 425 °F (220 °C) for 40 minutes or until mixture is set.

Yield: 8 servings
Exchange, 1 serving: ⅓ bread
½ fat
plus piecrust exchange
Calories, 1 serving: 64
plus piecrust calories

Coffee Chiffon Pie

The coffee is what makes it GOOD.

1 c.	skim evaporated milk	250 mL
½ c.	very strong coffee	125 mL
1 env.	unflavored gelatin	1 env.
¼ c.	cold water	60 mL
3	eggs separated	3
3 T.	granulated sugar replacement	45 mL
3 T.	cocoa	45 mL
⅛ t.	salt	½ mL
¼ t.	nutmeg	1 mL
½ t.	vanilla extract	2 mL
2 T.	chocolate sprinkles or jimmies	30 mL
9 in.	Basic Pie Shell, baked	23 cm

Scald milk and coffee. Sprinkle gelatin on cold water, allow to soften. Beat egg yolks, sugar replacement, cocoa, salt and nutmeg. Slowly add hot milk and coffee mixture. Add vanilla and softened gelatin. Chill until partially set. When mixture is partially set, beat well. Beat egg whites until stiff. Fold into cooled chocolate-coffee mixture. Pour into baked pie shell. Sprinkle top with chocolate sprinkles. Chill 2 to 3 hours or until firm.

Yield: 8 servings
Exchange, 1 serving: ⅓ bread
½ fat
plus piecrust exchange
Calories, 1 serving: 55
plus piecrust calories

Peanut Butter Pie

1¼ c.	hot water	60 mL
¼ c.	creamy peanut butter	60 mL
1 oz.	baking chocolate	30 g
¼ c.	sorbitol	60 mL
2 T.	granulated sugar replacement	30 mL
1¼ c.	skim evaporated milk	310 mL
3 T.	flour	45 mL
3 T.	cornstarch	45 mL
2	egg yolks, slightly beaten	2
1 t.	vanilla extract	5 mL
9 in.	Basic Pie Shell, baked	23 cm

Combine water, peanut butter and baking chocolate in top of double boiler. Cook and stir over simmering water until peanut butter and chocolate are melted. Stir in sorbitol and granulated sugar replacement. In a bowl, blend milk, flour and cornstarch together until smooth; gradually pour into chocolate mixture. Cook and stir until thickened. Pour small amount of chocolate mixture into beaten egg yolks and stir. Add egg mixture to pan. Cook and stir 2 minutes longer. Remove from heat; stir in vanilla. Cool slightly. Pour into baked pie shell. Chill in refrigerator until set, at least 2 hours.

Yield: 8 servings
Exchange, 1 serving: 1 high-fat meat
1 fat
½ fruit
plus piecrust exchange
Calories, 1 serving: 138
plus piecrust calories

White Raisin Pie

Thank you, Mrs. Danalo.

¾ c.	water	190 mL
¼ c.	semisweet chocolate chips	60 mL
1 c.	white raisins (sultanas)	250 mL
½ c.	skim evaporated milk	125 mL
1 t.	vanilla extract	5 mL
1 T.	granulated sugar replacement	15 mL
¼ c.	cornstarch	60 mL
⅛ t.	salt	½ mL
⅛ t.	cinnamon	½ mL
2	eggs	2
9 in.	Basic Pie Shell, unbaked	23 cm

Place water in heavy saucepan and bring to boil. Add chocolate chips and white raisins. Remove from heat, cover and allow to rest 15 minutes. Return to heat and add milk; warm slightly. Remove from heat and stir in vanilla extract. Mix together sugar replacement, cornstarch, salt and cinnamon. Stir into chocolate mixture. Beat eggs with electric mixer until frothy; stir into chocolate mixture. Pour into unbaked pie shell. Bake at 375 °F (190 °C) for 40 to 45 minutes or until set. Cool.

Yield: 8 servings
Exchange, 1 serving: 1½ bread
½ fat
plus piecrust exchange
Calories, 1 serving: 121
plus piecrust calories

Triple Decker Pie

Pretty and different—nice to serve.

9-in.	Chocolate Piecrust, unbaked	23 cm

Layer 1

2	eggs	2
¼ c.	milk chocolate chips, melted	60 mL
dash	salt	dash
1 t.	vanilla extract	5 mL
1 c.	skim milk	250 mL

Have the unbaked piecrust ready. Beat eggs in medium bowl until well blended. Add melted chocolate, salt, and vanilla extract. Beat one more minute. Stir in milk. Pour into pie shell. Bake at 300 °F (150 °C) for 50 minutes or until a knife inserted in center comes out clean. Cool.

Layer 2

1 c.	skim milk	250 mL
2 T.	flour	30 mL
1.5 oz.	baking chocolate	45 g
2 T.	sugar replacement	30 mL
2	egg yolks, slightly beaten	2
1 t.	vanilla extract	5 mL

Combine milk, flour, baking chocolate and sugar replacement in top of double boiler; cook and stir over medium heat until mixture thickens. Pour a small amount of chocolate mixture into egg yolks, then add to the large amount in the pan. Cook and stir until mixture is thick. Remove from heat and cover with waxed paper. When almost cool, remove paper and spread onto baked custard layer. Cool completely.

Layer 3

2 env.	unflavored gelatin	2 env.
¾ c.	water	190 mL
3 T.	sorbitol	45 mL

or

2 T.	granulated sugar replacement	30 mL
2 t.	white vanilla extract	10 mL
2	egg whites	2

In a saucepan, sprinkle gelatin over water, allow to soften for 5 minutes. Place pan over medium heat and bring to a boil. Cook until gelatin is dissolved. Remove from heat, add sorbitol and white vanilla. Stir to blend completely. Allow to cool until mixture is consistency of thick syrup. Beat egg whites into soft peaks. With a slow stream, add gelatin mixture, beating constantly into stiff peaks. Spread over entire surface of pie. Chill until firm.

Yield: 8 servings
Exchange, 1 serving: 1 high-fat meat
1 fruit
½ fat
plus piecrust exchange
Calories, 1 serving: 125
plus piecrust calories

Pecan Chocolate-Chip Pie

½ c.	butter, softened	125 mL
2 T.	granulated sugar replacement	30 mL
3	eggs	3
1 t.	vanilla extract	5 mL
1 T.	flour	15 mL
⅓ c.	semisweet chocolate chips	90 mL
¼ c.	pecans, chopped	60 mL
10 in.	Basic Pie Shell, unbaked	25 cm

Cream butter and sugar replacement in large bowl until fluffy. Beat in eggs and vanilla extract. Add flour and blend until smooth; fold in chocolate chips and pecans. Pour mixture into unbaked pie shell. Bake at 325 °F (165 °C) for about 50 minutes or until center is set and top is golden.

Yield: 8 servings
Exchange, 1 serving: 1 high-fat meat
3 fat
½ fruit
plus piecrust exchange
Calories, 1 serving: 220
plus piecrust calories

Perfection Pie

3 T.	chocolate chips	45 mL
⅓ c.	water, boiling	90 mL
3	eggs	3
1 T.	cornstarch	15 mL
3 T.	granulated sugar replacement	45 mL
2 T.	vegetable shortening, melted	30 mL
8 in.	Basic Pie Shell, unbaked	20 cm

Melt chocolate chips in boiling water; set aside to cool. Beat eggs; blend in cornstarch and sugar replacement. Continue beating and add the shortening and, gradually, the chocolate mixture. Pour into pie shell. Bake at 400°F (200 °C) for about 35 minutes or until custard is set.

Yield: 8 servings
Exchange, 1 serving: ⅓ bread
1 fat
plus piecrust exchange
Calories, 1 serving: 86
plus piecrust calories

French Silk Pie

If I'm going to "blow" calories, this is the one!

1 oz.	baking chocolate	30 g
⅓ c.	sweet butter	90 mL
6 pkg.	aspartame sweetener	6 pkg.
1 t.	vanilla extract	5 mL
2	eggs	2
8 in.	Basic Pie Shell, baked	20 cm

Melt chocolate in top of double boiler; cool. Cream butter with aspartame sweetener until light and fluffy. Blend in chocolate and vanilla. Add eggs, one at a time, beating 5 minutes after each addition, using medium speed on electric mixer. Turn into baked pie shell and chill at least 1 to 2 hours before serving.

Yield: 8 servings
Exchange, 1 serving: 2⅕ fat
plus piecrust exchange
Calories, 1 serving: 110
plus piecrust calories

Brownie Pie

3	eggs	3
1/4 c.	margarine	60 mL
5 T.	sorbitol	75 mL
3 T.	granulated sugar replacement	45 mL
3/4 c.	flour	190 mL
1/2 t.	salt	2 mL
2 oz.	baking chocolate, melted	60 g
1/3 c.	skim milk	90 mL
1 t.	vanilla extract	5 mL

Beat eggs until very light and thickened. Cream margarine; gradually add sorbitol and sugar replacement, beating until light and fluffy. Sift together the flour and salt; set aside. Add cooled baking chocolate and beaten eggs to creamed margarine mixture. Alternately add the flour and milk to creamed mixture. Add vanilla. Pour into a greased 9-in. (23-cm) pie pan. Bake at 375°F (190 °C) for 45 to 50 minutes or until pie tests done.

Yield: 8 servings
Exchange, 1 serving: ½ medium-fat meat
  1 fat
  1 fruit
  plus piecrust exchange
Calories, 1 serving: 121
  plus piecrust calories

Chip Pie

30	Marshmallows	30
1 c.	skim milk	250 mL
1 oz.	baking chocolate	30 g
1 env.	low-cal topping mix	1 env.
1 t.	vanilla	5 mL
9 in.	Crumb Piecrust Shell (made with graham crackers)	23 cm

Melt marshmallows in ½ c. (125 mL) milk in double boiler. Stir constantly. Cool over pan of cold water. Chip or grate the chocolate into small pieces and add to marshmallow mixture. Add vanilla and the remaining ½ c. (125 mL) skim milk to the topping mix. Beat into stiff peaks. Fold into cooled marshmallow mixture. Pour into graham cracker shell. Chill at least 2 hours before serving.

Yield: 8 servings
Exchange, 1 serving: ½ low-fat milk
plus piecrust exchange
Calories, 1 serving: 49
plus piecrust calories

Basic Pie Shell

⅓ c.	vegetable shortening	90 mL
1 c.	flour, sifted	250 mL
¼ t.	salt	1 mL
2 to 4 T.	ice water	30 to 60 mL

Chill shortening. Cut shortening into flour and salt until mixture forms crumbs. Add ice water, 1 T. (15 mL) at a time, and flip mixture around in bowl until a ball forms. Wrap ball in plastic wrap and chill at least 1 hour. Roll to fit 9-in. (23-cm) pie pan. Fill with pie filling or prick with fork. Bake at 425 °F (220 °C) for 10 to 12 minutes or until firm. Or leave unbaked and refrigerate or freeze until ready to use.

Yield: 8 servings
Exchange, 1 serving: 1 bread
1 fat
Calories, 1 serving: 120

Chocolate Piecrust

¾ c.	flour	190 mL
3 T.	cocoa	45 mL
⅓ c.	vegetable shortening, softened	90 mL
1 t.	liquid fructose	5 mL

or

1 T.	granulated sugar replacement	15 mL
2 to 3 T.	cold water	30 to 45 mL

In a food processor or bowl, combine flour, cocoa, shortening and fructose; work into crumbs. Add enough water to make a soft ball. Roll up or press into sides and bottom on pie pan. Use as directed in recipe.

Yield: 8 servings
Exchange, 1 serving: ¾ bread
2 fat
Calories, 1 serving: 129

Crumb Piecrust Shell

1¼ c.	graham cracker or zwieback crumbs, finely crushed	310 mL
3 T.	margarine, melted	45 mL
1 T.	water	15 mL

Combine crumbs with melted margarine and water. Spread dough evenly in 8-to 10-in. (20- to 25-cm) pie pan, pressing firmly onto sides and bottom. Either chill until set, or bake at 325 °F (165 °C) for 8 to 10 minutes

Yield: 8 servings
Exchange, 1 serving graham cracker crumbs: 1 bread
1 fat
Calories, 1 serving graham cracker crumbs: 85
Exchange, 1 serving dry cereal crumbs: ½ bread
1 fat
Calories, 1 serving dry cereal crumbs: 64
Exchange, 1 serving zwieback crumbs: ½ bread
1 fat
Calories, 1 serving zwieback crumbs: 70

Chilled Desserts

Easy Chocolate Ice Cream

½ c.	skim milk	125 mL
¼ c.	semisweet chocolate chips	60 mL
1 env.	nondairy topping mix	1 env.

Heat milk and chocolate chips just to boiling, stirring constantly to dissolve chips. Refrigerate until mixture is very cold. Add topping mix. Beat until mixture is thick and fluffy. Pour into freezer box or tray and freeze until firm.

Yield: 2 c. (500 mL)
Exchange, ½ c. (125 mL): 1 bread
⅗ fat
Calories, ½ c. (125 mL): 97

Ice Cream Clones

1 recipe	Easy Chocolate Ice Cream	1 recipe
20	Cream Puff Pastry Mini Cream Puffs	20

Prepare Easy Chocolate Ice Cream but **do not freeze**. Scoop mixture into pastry bag with a large tube. Squeeze mixture into the mini cream puffs. Freeze.

Yield: 20 clones
Exchange, 1 clone: ⅓ bread
Calories, 1 clone: 21

Chocolate Mint Gelatin

A lean and flavorful dessert.

¼ c.	cocoa	60 mL
3 T.	granulated sugar replacement	45 mL
1 env.	unflavored gelatin	1 env.
1 c.	boiling water	250 mL
½ c.	plain nonfat yogurt	125 mL
2 t.	mint extract	10 mL
½ t.	vanilla extract	2 mL
½ c.	cold water ·	125 mL
1 c.	nondairy whipped topping	250 mL

Combine cocoa, sugar replacement, and gelatin in medium-sized mixing bowl. Stir to mix. Pour boiling water over mixture and stir to completely dissolve ingredients. Stir in yogurt, extracts and cold water. Pour into 2 c. (500 mL) decorative mould. Chill until set. Unmould and decorate with nondairy whipped topping.

Yield: 6 servings
Exchange, 1 serving: ½ no-fat milk
Calories, 1 serving: 48

Mocha Dessert

½ c.	chocolate chips	125 mL
2 c.	hot coffee	500 mL
1 env.	unflavored gelatin	1 env.
1 env.	nondairy topping mix	1 env.

In a medium-sized mixing bowl, dissolve the chocolate chips and gelatin in the hot coffee. Cool. Stir in nondairy whipped topping powder until it is completely blended. Place mixing bowl in a larger bowl of ice. Beat with a whip or electric mixer until mixture is slightly fluffy. Divide into 8 sherbet or dessert glasses. Chill until completely set.

Yield: 8 servings
Exchange, 1 serving: ⅔ bread
1 fat
Calories, 1 serving: 71

Split Parfaits

No one can resist these.

2 c.	*fresh strawberries*	*500 mL*
2 T.	*sorbitol*	*30 mL*
2 c.	*Easy Chocolate Ice Cream*	*500 mL*
1½	*bananas, sliced*	*1½*

Mash strawberries. Stir in sorbitol and set aside for 20 minutes. Place 2 T. (30 mL) of mashed strawberries in bottom of 6 parfait glasses. Add ⅓ c. (90 mL) of ice cream and ⅙ of banana slices to glasses. Top each glass with equal amounts of remaining strawberries.

Yield: 6 servings
Exchange, 1 serving: ⅔ bread
1 fruit
⅓ fat
Calories, 1 serving: 108

Sweet Chocolate Turban

2 env.	*unflavored gelatin*	2
½ c.	*cold water*	*125 mL*
⅓ c.	*granulated sugar replacement*	*90 mL*
2 T.	*liquid fructose*	*30 mL*
½ c.	*chocolate chips*	*125 mL*
2½ c.	*buttermilk*	*625 mL*
1 c.	*Chocolate Whipped Topping*	*250 mL*

Sprinkle the gelatin on top of cold water in a saucepan. Allow to soften for 5 minutes. Cook and stir over low heat until the gelatin is completely dissolved. Remove from heat and add sugar replacement, fructose and chocolate chips. Stir until blended. Stir in buttermilk. Mix thoroughly. Pour into a lightly greased turban mould or decorative ice cream mould. Refrigerate until firm, about 3 to 4 hours. Unmould onto a well-chilled serving plate. Decorate around the edge with chocolate whipped topping.

Yield: 6 servings
Exchange, 1 serving: 1 bread
1 fat
Calories, 1 serving: 117

Chocolate Pecan Gelatin

¼ c.	pecans	60 mL
1 env.	unflavored gelatin	1 env.
1 c.	cold water	250 mL
3 T.	granulated sugar replacement	45 mL
3 T.	cocoa	45 mL
dash	salt	dash
1 c.	skim milk	250 mL

Chop pecans and lightly toast. Set aside. Sprinkle gelatin over cold water and allow to soften for 5 minutes. In a microwave or on top of the stove bring mixture to boiling. Remove from heat. Add sugar replacement, cocoa and salt. Whip to thoroughly mix. Stir in skim milk. Allow to cool and set to consistency of thick syrup. Fold in toasted pecans. Turn into 4 dessert dishes. Chill.

Yield: 4 servings
Exchange, 1 serving: ⅓ fat
                    1 fat
Calories, 1 serving: 86

Holiday Treat

1 env.	low-cal chocolate pudding mix	1 env.
2 c.	skim milk	500 mL
1 t.	orange flavoring	5 mL
8	no-sugar pear halves	8
2 t.	walnuts, finely ground	10 mL

Combine pudding mix and skim milk in saucepan. Bring to boil over low heat, stir constantly. Remove from heat and cool slightly. Stir in orange flavoring. Place pear halves in individual serving dishes. Top with equal amounts of pudding mixture. Sprinkle lightly with ¼ t. (1 mL) finely ground walnuts. Refrigerate until thoroughly chilled.

Yield: 8 servings
Exchange, 1 serving: 1 no-fat milk
                    1 fruit
Calories, 1 serving: 112

Mocha Ice Cream

A bittersweet treat.

2	eggs	2
2	egg yolks	2
3 T.	granulated sugar replacement	45 mL
2 T.	sorbitol	30 mL
2 c.	milk (2% fat)	500 mL
1 T.	cornstarch	15 mL
2 oz.	baking chocolate, melted	60 g
2 T.	very strong coffee	30 mL
1 c.	nondairy whipped topping	250 mL

Beat egg and egg yolks in bowl; add sugar replacement and sorbitol and beat until thick and creamy. Combine milk and cornstarch in saucepan; stir to thoroughly mix. Heat until mixture is about to boil and is slightly thickened. Remove from heat and pour over egg mixture in a steady stream. Beat thoroughly to blend. Return mixture to saucepan, cook and stir over low heat until custard thickens. (DO NOT ALLOW TO BOIL.) Stir in melted chocolate and strong coffee. Place hot saucepan in bowl over ice cubes, to speed the cooling process. When cool to the touch, fold in whipped topping. Chill and freeze. As it hardens, push the sides of the mixture to the center. When nearly set, scrape mixture into large mixing bowl. Beat well. Pack and freeze.

Yield: 8 servings
Exchange, 1 serving: ½ bread
⅔ high-fat meat
Calories, 1 serving: 122

Frozen Chocolate Banana Yogurt

Quick and easy.

1	very ripe banana	1
2 T.	cocoa	30 mL
8 oz.	plain yogurt	226 g

Combine banana, cocoa and yogurt in blender or food processor. Blend until smooth. Turn into two dessert dishes. Freeze until firm.

Yield: 2 servings:
Exchange: 1 no-fat milk
⅔ bread
Calories: 132

Chocolate Bavarian Dessert

1 env.	unflavored gelatin	1 env.
2 T.	cold water	30 mL
4	egg yolks	4
2 T.	granulated sugar replacement	30 mL
1 T.	liquid fructose	15 mL
1 c.	skim milk	250 mL
1 oz.	baking chocolate	30 g
1 t.	brandy flavoring	5 mL
1 c.	nondairy whipped topping	250 mL

Soak the gelatin in the cold water; set aside. In the top of a double boiler beat the egg yolks, sugar replacement and fructose until smooth and thick. Heat skim milk with the baking chocolate until chocolate is melted and milk is hot **but not boiling**. Gradually beat milk mixture into the egg mixture. Cook and stir over simmering water until custard is smooth and thickened. Set aside to cool slightly. Stir in softened gelatin and brandy flavoring; mix thoroughly. Cool the custard, stirring occasionally to prevent the formation of a skin. When the custard is cooled, fold in the nondairy whipped topping. Turn into a chilled 1-qt. (1-L) mould. Refrigerate for several hours before unmoulding onto a serving platter.

Yield: 10 servings
Exchange, 1 serving: ⅓ bread
1 fat
Calories, 1 serving: 59

Cool Chocolate Gelatin

A fast perfection while you do other chores.

1 env.	unflavored gelatin	1 env.
½ c.	cold water	125 mL
1½ c.	chocolate milk (2% fat)	375 mL

Sprinkle gelatin over water; allow to soften for 5 minutes. In microwave or on top of the stove bring mixture to boiling. Allow to cool slightly. Stir in chocolate milk. Pour into 4 dessert dishes. Chill.

Yield: 4 servings
Exchange, 1 serving: ⅔ low-fat milk
Calories, 1 serving: 70

Cool Chocolate Custard Ice Cream

4	egg yolks	4
3 T.	granulated sugar replacement	45 mL
1 c.	milk (2% fat)	250 mL
2 oz.	baking chocolate, melted	60 g
2 c.	nondairy whipped topping	500 mL

In a medium-sized mixing bowl beat the egg yolks with the sugar replacement until light and fluffy. Heat milk just to boiling. Pour hot milk over egg yolk mixture, beating constantly. Beat in melted chocolate. Return mixture to saucepan. Cook and stir over low heat until mixture thickens. Remove from heat and cool. Beat slightly with electric mixture to loosen. Fold prepared nondairy whipped topping into custard. Chill or freeze.

Yield: 8 servings
Exchange, 1 serving: ⅔ low-fat milk
                        1 fat
Calories, 1 serving: 112

Spanish Delight

1	cinnamon stick	1
¼ t.	ground nutmeg	2 mL
dash	ground cloves	dash
dash	ground ginger	dash
2 c.	water	500 mL
1 env.	unflavored gelatin	1 env.
½ c.	chocolate chips	125 mL
3 T.	granulated sugar replacement	45 mL

Combine cinnamon stick, nutmeg, cloves and ginger with water in saucepan. Bring to a boil, reduce heat and simmer for 5 minutes. Remove from heat. Remove cinnamon stick. Add unflavored gelatin, chocolate chips and sugar replacement. Stir to dissolve completely. Refrigerate until completely set.

Yield: 4 servings
Exchange, 1 serving: 1 bread
                        1 fat
Calories, 1 serving: 110

Fudge Almandine Mousse

6	egg yolks	6
3 T.	liquid fructose	45 mL
2 c.	nondairy whipped topping	500 mL
7	egg whites	7
1/3 c.	almonds, toasted and ground	90 mL
1/2 c.	chocolate chips, ground	125 mL
1 T.	rum flavoring	15 mL

Beat egg yolks until pale and creamy. Pour liquid fructose over yolks and beat until thick. Fold in nondairy whipped topping. Beat egg whites and salt until stiff. Fold into mixture. Fold in ground almonds and chocolate chips. Pile into decorate mould and freeze. Allow to soften 15 minutes in refrigerator before unmoulding. Unmould onto serving plate. Sprinkle with rum flavoring.

Yield: 10 servings
Exchange, 1 serving: 2/3 high-fat meat
1 fruit
Calories, 1 serving: 125

Chocolate Yogurt Ice

3 c.	crushed ice	750 mL
8 oz.	plain nonfat yogurt	226 g
2 oz.	baking chocolate, melted	60 g
3 T.	granulated sugar replacement	45 mL
4 T.	nondairy whipped topping	60 mL

Combine all ingredients in food processor or blender. Whip until thoroughly blended but not melted. Pour into 4 tall glasses. Place in freezer until mixture is slightly frozen. Stir, top with 1 T. (15 mL) nondairy whipped topping and serve.

Yield: 4 servings
Exchange, 1 serving: 1/5 full-fat milk
Calories, 1 serving: 134

Chocolate Buttermilk Ice

A German specialty.

1 qt.	buttermilk	1 L
2 oz.	baking chocolate, melted	60 g
3 T.	granulated sugar replacement	45 mL

Mix all ingredients thoroughly in a large mixing bowl. Pour into a freezer tray or metal baking dish. Freeze until mushy and slightly frozen around the edges of the tray. Return to large mixing bowl and beat until the mixture is light. Pile into 6 individual sherbet dishes and freeze until ready to serve.

Yield: 6 servings
Exchange, 1 serving: 1 medium-fat milk
Calories, 1 serving: 116

Christmas Dessert

An elegant dessert. Make it in advance.

4	egg yolks	4
⅓ c.	granulated sugar replacement	90 mL
1 T.	crème de cacao	15 mL
4	egg whites	4
⅓ c.	pecans, finely ground	90 mL
1 env.	nondairy topping mix	1 env.
½ c.	skim milk	125 mL
3 drops	green food coloring	3 drops

Cook egg yolks, sugar replacement and crème de cacao over low heat in the top of a double boiler until thick; cool. Beat egg whites until stiff. Fold egg whites into cooled custard mixture. Fold in chopped pecans. Beat topping mix with skim milk and green food coloring until stiff. Fold into custard mixture. Turn into well-chilled 1½-qt. (1½-L) serving dish. Refrigerate or freeze. If frozen, allow to set at room temperature 15 minutes before serving.

Yield: 10 servings
Exchange, 1 serving: ½ high-fat meat
½ fruit
Calories, 1 serving: 73

Chocolate Chip Walnut Ice Cream

1	egg	1
1	egg yolk	1
2 T.	granulated sugar replacement	30 mL
1 c.	whole milk	250 mL
2 t.	cornstarch	10 mL
1 c.	nondairy whipped topping	250 mL
1/3 c.	mini chocolate chips	90 mL
1/3 c.	walnuts, chopped	90 mL

Beat egg, egg yolk and sugar replacement until thick and smooth. Combine milk and cornstarch in top of double boiler and stir and cook over simmering water until slightly thickened. Add small amount of milk mixture to egg mixture; stir to blend. Return to saucepan. Continue stirring and cooking until mixture is thick. Cool to room temperature. Beat well with electric mixer. Fold in prepared nondairy whipped topping. Fold in chocolate chips and walnuts. Pack and freeze.

Yield: 6 servings
Exchange, 1 serving: 2/3 full-fat milk
Calories, 1 serving: 156

Pineapple au Chocolat

Something for one.

2	pineapple slices, drained	2
1	large lettuce leaf	1
2 T.	Chocolate Topping	30 mL
1 T.	nondairy whipped topping	15 mL

Place pineapple slices on lettuce leaf, drizzle with chocolate topping. Top with whipped topping.

Yield: 1 serving:
Exchange: 2/3 bread
*   1 fruit*
Calories: 88

Chocolate Bombe

1 recipe	Easy Chocolate Ice Cream	1 recipe
1 c.	vanilla ice cream	250 mL
1 c.	nondairy whipped topping	250 mL
¼ c.	almonds, toasted and finely chopped	60 mL

Chill a 1-qt. (1-L) metal mould in the freezer. With a chilled spoon, quickly spread chocolate ice cream over bottom and sides of mould. Freeze firm. Stir the vanilla ice cream just to soften. Quickly spread over chocolate layer, covering completely. Freeze firm. Fold toasted almonds into whipped topping. Pile into center of mould, smoothing the top. Cover with plastic wrap or foil. Freeze 6 to 8 hours or overnight. Peel off cover, invert mould onto chilled plate. Cover mould with a damp warm towel; lift off mould. Refreeze or serve.

Yield: 14 servings
Exchange, 1 serving: ½ bread
                    ⅔ fat
Calories, 1 serving: 65

Syrups, Beverages, Toppings and Frostings

Low-low-Cal Syrup

1 env.	*unflavored gelatin*	*1 env.*
2½ c.	*water*	*625 mL*
2 T.	*cocoa*	*30 mL*
3 pkg.	*aspartame sweetener*	*3 pkg.*

Sprinkle gelatin over water in saucepan and allow to soften for 5 minutes. Bring to boil and stir in cocoa. Allow to cool. Add aspartame and stir to completely dissolve. Place in refrigerator. Stir occasionally to keep cocoa in suspension.

Yield: 2 c. (500 mL)
Exchange, full recipe: 1 bread
1 fat
Calories, full recipe: 120
For a richer sauce, add ½ c. (125 mL) dry milk powder

Yield: 2 c. (500 mL)
Exchange, full recipe: ½ bread
2 no-fat milk
1 fat
Calories, full recipe: 240

Old-Fashioned Hot Chocolate

2 oz.	baking chocolate	60 g
1 c.	water	250 mL
dash	salt	dash
3 c.	skim milk	750 mL
2 T.	liquid sugar replacement	30 mL

Cook chocolate and water over low heat until chocolate is melted. Add salt and cook for 2 minutes. Gradually stir in milk and stir constantly. When mixture is piping hot, remove from heat and add liquid sugar replacement. Beat until frothy. Serve in warmed mugs.

Yield: 4 servings
Exchange, 1 serving: ¾ no-fat milk
                    2 fat
Calories, 1 serving: 130

Cinnamon-Chocolate Drink

Perfect to drink on a cold, winter night.

4 c.	skim milk	1 L
2 oz.	semisweet chocolate	60 g
2	cinnamon sticks	2
1 t.	vanilla	5 mL

Combine milk, semisweet chocolate and cinnamon sticks in saucepan. Cook and stir over low heat until chocolate melts. Remove from heat and stir in vanilla. Remove cinnamon sticks. Serve in warmed mugs.

Yield: 4 servings
Exchange, 1 serving: 1 high-fat milk
Calories, 1 serving: 170

Instant Drink Mix

2 c.	dry milk	500 mL
¼ c.	cocoa	60 mL
4 pkg.	aspartame sweetener	4 pkg.

Combine all ingredients in electric blender. Blend at high speed to thoroughly mix.

Cold: Pour ice water into a tall glass. Add 3 T. (45 mL) instant drink mix and stir briskly to dissolve completely.

Hot: Place 3 T. (45 mL) of instant drink mix in a cup. Add hot water and stir to dissolve.

Yield: 1½ c. (375 mL)
Exchange, 3 T. (45 mL): ¾ low-fat milk
Calories, 3 T. (45 mL): 62
  If milk is used, add milk exchange and calories.

Instant Chocolate Syrup

1	Instant Drink Mix	1
1 c.	hot water	250 mL

Combine ingredients and stir to dissolve completely. Chill or use hot.

Yield: 1 c. (250 mL)
Exchange: 6 low-fat milk
Calories: 480

Instant Banana Shake

1	ripe banana	1
3 T.	Instant Drink Mix	45 mL
1 c.	milk (2% fat)	250 mL

Slice banana into a bowl and beat until creamy. Beat in drink mix. Add milk and mix thoroughly. Serve at once.

Yield: 2 servings
Exchange, 1 serving: ¾ low-fat milk
                    1 fruit
Calories, 1 serving: 143

Instant Ice Cream Soda

So-o-o-o good.

3 T.	Instant Drink Mix	45 mL
¼ c.	cold water	60 mL
½ c.	vanilla ice cream, softened	125 mL
½ can	cold diet soda	½ can

Combine drink mix and water in a tall glass, stir to completely blend. Add ice cream and fill with diet soda.

Yield: 1 serving
Exchange: 1 bread
            1 low-fat milk
Calories: 200

Mocha Drink

1 c.	water	250 mL
2 T.	instant coffee	30 mL
2 oz.	baking chocolate	60 g
dash	salt	dash
3 c.	skim milk	750 mL
5 pkg.	granulated sugar replacement	5 pkg.

Combine water, instant coffee, baking chocolate and salt in saucepan. Cook and stir over low heat until chocolate melts. Gradually add milk, stirring constantly. When piping hot, remove from heat. Stir in sugar replacement. Serve in cups or mugs. (Optional: Top each cup with 1 T. (15 mL) prepared nondairy whipped topping.)

Yield: 4 servings
Exchange, 1 serving: ¾ no-fat milk
                    2 fat
Calories: 1 serving: 130
Exchange, 1 serving with topping: ⅓ no-fat milk
                                2 fat
Calories: 1 serving with topping: 138

Crème de Cacao-Cola

My personal favorite after-dinner drink.

1 T.	crème de cacao	15 mL
3/4 c.	diet cola soda	190 mL
	ice	

Combine all ingredients in glass, stir to blend.

Yield: 1 drink
Exchange: 1/5 bread
Calories: 15

Chocolate Drizzle

2 t.	cornstarch	10 mL
1/4 c.	cold water	60 mL
dash	salt	dash
1 oz.	baking chocolate	30 g
1/3 c.	granulated sugar replacement	90 mL
1/2 t.	butter	3 mL

Blend cornstarch and cold water and pour into small saucepan. Add salt and chocolate. Cook on low heat until chocolate melts and mixture is thick; remove from heat. Stir in sugar replacement and blend in butter. Use over cake or ice cream.

Yield: 1/3 c. (90 mL)
Exchange: negligible
Calories: negligible

Chocolate Topping

3 c.	skim milk	750 mL
2 oz.	baking chocolate	60 g
3 T.	cornstarch	45 mL
½ c.	granulated sugar replacement	125 mL
1 t.	salt	5 mL
2 T.	butter	30 mL
2 t.	vanilla extract	10 mL

Combine milk, chocolate, cornstarch, sugar replacement and salt in saucepan. Bring to a full boil, and boil for 2 to 3 minutes; remove from heat. Stir in the butter and vanilla.

Yield: 3 c. (750 mL)
Exchange, 2 T. (30 mL): ½ fat
Calories, 2 T. (30 mL): 35

Chocolate Eggnog

1	egg, beaten (see note below)	1
3 T.	Chocolate Topping	45 mL
dash	salt	dash
¾ c.	skim milk	190 mL
¼ t.	vanilla extract	2 mL

Combine all ingredients in tall glass or mixing bowl. Beat to blend. Serve at once.

Yield: 1 serving
Exchange, 1 serving: 1 medium-fat meat
¾ medium-fat milk
Calories, 1 serving: 175

Note: For a creamier eggnog: Separate egg and beat yolk with all the ingredients. Beat egg white separately until stiff. Then fold egg white into eggnog mixture.

Chocolate Marshmallow Frosting

2 env.	unflavored gelatin	2 env.
¾ c.	water	190 mL
3 T.	cocoa	45 mL
3 T.	granulated sugar replacement	45 mL
1 T.	white vanilla extract	15 mL
2	egg whites	2

Sprinkle gelatin over water in saucepan; allow to soften for 5 minutes. Cook and stir over medium heat until gelatin is dissolved. Remove from heat and cool to the consistency of thick syrup. Add cocoa, sugar replacement and vanilla, stirring to blend. Beat egg whites into soft peaks. Very slowly, trickle a small stream of gelatin mixture into egg whites, beat until all gelatin mixture is blended. Continue beating until light and fluffy.

Yield: Frosts sides and tops of two 9-in. (23-cm) layers or one 9 × 13-in. (23 × 33-cm) cake or 30 cupcakes.
Exchange, 1 serving: negligible
Calories, 1 serving: negligible

Nut Frosting

A frosting which complements all cakes.

1	egg	1
⅓ c.	granulated brown sugar replacement	90 mL
2 t.	vanilla extract	10 mL
⅓ c.	semisweet chocolate chips	90 mL
½ c.	walnuts, chopped	125 mL

Combine egg, brown sugar replacement and vanilla in bowl. Beat with an electric mixer until thick. Stir in chocolate chips and walnuts. Spoon and spread over hot cake or cupcakes. Place in 350 °F (175 °C) oven for 10 minutes. Remove and cool.

Yield: 24 servings
Exchange, 1 serving: ⅗ fat
Calories, 1 serving: 31

Chocolate Whipped Topping

1 env.	nondairy topping mix	1 env.
2 T.	cocoa	30 mL
dash	salt	dash
½ t.	vanilla extract	2 mL
½ c.	ice water	125 mL
2 T.	Powdered Sugar Replacement	30 mL

Combine topping mix, cocoa and salt in mixing bowl; stir to blend. Add vanilla and water, and beat until soft peaks form. Gradually, add sugar replacement and beat until mixture is stiff.

Yield: 2 c. (500 mL)
Exchange, 1 T. (15 mL): negligible
Calories, 1 T. (15 mL): 11

Cocoan Frosting

I developed "cocoan" by combining coconut and pecans (ingredients and letters).

1	egg	1
⅓ c.	granulated brown sugar replacement	90 mL
1 t.	vanilla extract	5 mL
⅓ c.	unsweetened coconut, grated	90 mL
⅓ c.	pecans, finely chopped	90 mL

Combine egg, brown sugar replacement and vanilla in bowl. Beat with an electric mixer until thick. Stir in coconut and pecans. Spoon and spread over cake. Bake in a 350 °F (175 °C) oven for 10 minutes.

Yield: 24 servings
Exchange, 1 serving: ⅓ fat
Calories, 1 serving: 18

Smooth-As-Silk Frosting

1 env.	unflavored gelatin	1 env.
1/2 c.	water	125 mL
1/3 c.	granulated brown sugar replacement	90 mL
2	egg whites, stiffly beaten	2
1 t.	vanilla extract	5 mL

Sprinkle gelatin over water in saucepan; allow to soften for 5 minutes. Bring to a boil. Add brown sugar replacement and stir to dissolve. Remove from heat; cool to the consistency of thin syrup. Beating constantly, pour syrup in a thin stream into beaten egg whites. Beat in vanilla.

Yield: Frosts sides and tops of any size cake.
Exchange, 1 serving: negligible
Calories, 1 serving: negligible

Cherry Yogurt Frosting

1	egg white	1
2 T.	cherry yogurt	30 mL

Beat egg white to soft peaks; gradually add the yogurt. Beat to stiff peaks. Spread on 8- or 9-in. (20- or 23-cm) cake. Serve immediately.

Yield: 9 servings
Exchange, 1 serving: negligible
Calories, 1 serving: negligible

Caramel Fluff Frosting

1 env.	nondairy topping mix	1 env.
1/2 c.	skim milk	125 mL
1/4 c.	granulated brown sugar replacement	60 mL
1 t.	vanilla extract	5 mL

Combine all ingredients in a chilled bowl. Beat into stiff peaks.

Yield: 2 c. (500 mL) or 20 servings
Exchange, 1 serving: 1/2 bread
Calories, 1 serving: 9

Plain Chocolate Frosting

1 c.	skim evaporated milk	250 mL
2 T.	cornstarch	30 mL
¼ c.	granulated sugar replacement	60 mL
2 oz.	baking chocolate, melted	60 g
1 t.	vanilla extract	5 mL
dash	salt	dash
3 T.	water	45 mL

Combine all ingredients in top of double boiler. Cook, stirring constantly, over boiling water until thick. Cool. Beat to spreading consistency.

Yield: Frosts 9 × 13-in. (23 × 33-cm) cake or 24 servings
Exchange, 1 serving: ⅓ bread
⅓ fat
Calories, 1 serving: 25

Crème Semisweet Chocolate Frosting

¼ c.	semisweet chocolate chips	60 mL
2 T.	butter	30 mL
¼ c.	skim evaporated milk	60 mL
½ recipe	Marshmallow Crème	½ recipe

Melt chocolate chips and butter in top of double boiler over boiling water. Gradually add evaporated milk and stir until smooth. Allow to cool to room temperature. Add marshmallow crème and beat until smooth.

Yield: Frosts sides and tops of 8- or 9-in. (20- or 23-cm) layer cake
Exchange, ⅟₂₀ of cake: ½ fat
Calories, ⅟₂₀ of cake: 23
Exchange, ⅟₂₄ of cake: ⅔ fat
Calories, ⅟₂₄ of cake: 19

Appendix

Food Exchange Lists

Your Diet and the Big Six

A diabetic's diet is multipurpose. First, it is to keep you in good health and, second, to keep the disease under control. Perhaps it would be easier to understand the individual nutritional needs if we understood what happens to food after it is swallowed. The body uses the three energy elements from food to: 1) develop heat and energy from carbohydrates; 2) develop new muscle and blood tissue from protein; 3) develop protective covering for organs from fat. Because the diabetic cannot digest and metabolize food the same way the non-diabetic can, the American Diabetes Association has developed an "Exchange List" for foods.*

The Exchange Lists are grouped into six basic food groups: milk, vegetable, fruit, bread, meat, and fat. Food in any one group or exchange may be substituted for any other food in the same group or exchange; all foods within the same group or exchange have approximately the same grams of carbohydrates, proteins, fats and calorie values. By picking and choosing from the Exchange List, it's easy to develop meals that are both tasty and appealing to you as an individual.

*The exchange lists are based on material in the *Exchange Lists for Meal Planning* prepared by Committees of the American Diabetes Association, Inc., and the American Dietetic Association in cooperation with the National Institute of Arthritis, Metabolism and Digestive Diseases and the National Heart and Lung Institutes of Health, Public Health Service, U.S. Department of Health and Human Services.

Suppose your doctor or diet counsellor has told you that for breakfast you should have the following exchanges:

1 fruit
2 bread
2 meat
1 milk
1 fat

By referring to the Exchange List, you could make up a breakfast something like this:

4 oz. (125 mL) orange juice	1 fruit
1 toasted English muffin	2 bread
2 eggs	2 meat
8 oz. (250 mL) milk	1 milk
1 t. (5 mL) margarine or butter	1 fat
or	
½ grapefruit	1 fruit
¾ c. (190 mL) puffed or flaked cereal	1 bread
1 piece of toast	1 bread
2 oz. (60 g) Canadian bacon	2 meat
8 oz. (250 mL) milk	1 milk
1 t. (5 mL) margarine or butter	1 fat
or	
¼ cantaloupe	1 fruit
1 c. (250 mL) cooked rice	2 bread
2 oz. (60 g) pork sausage	2 meat
8 oz. (250 mL) milk	1 milk
1 t. (5 mL) margarine or butter	1 fat
or	
¾ c. (190 mL) strawberries blended with 1 c. (250 mL) yogurt	1 fruit 1 milk
Small cheese omelette	2 meat
2 pieces of toast	2 bread
1 t. (5 mL) margarine or butter	1 fat

As you can see, there is a wide selection open to you. When you start planning your meals, remember to ask your doctor or diet counsellor if you have any questions—never guess on your own.

Milk Exchange

Nonfat: One exchange contains 12 grams carbohydrates, 8 grams protein, and 80 calories.

Nonfat milk (skim, buttermilk, plain yogurt)	1 c. (250 mL)
Nonfat canned	½ c. (125 mL)
Nonfat powdered solids	⅓ c. (90 mL)

Low-fat: One exchange contains 12 grams carbohydrates, 8 grams protein, 5 grams fat, and 125 calories.

1%; omit ½ fat exchange	1 c. (250 mL)
2% milk; omit 1 fat exchange	1 c. (250 mL)
2% yogurt; omit 1 fat exchange	1 c. (250 mL)

Full-fat: One exchange contains 12 grams carbohydrates, 8 grams protein, 10 grams fat, and 170 calories; omit 2 fat exchanges.

Whole milk, buttermilk, plain yogurt	1 c. (250 mL)
Canned whole milk	½ c. (125 mL)

Vegetable Exchange

One exchange, cooked without fat, contains 5 grams carbohydrates, 2 grams protein and 25 calories. One exchange is ½ c. (125 mL), cooked.

Asparagus	Mushrooms
Bamboo shoots	Onions
Bean sprouts	Rutabaga
Broccoli	Sauerkraut
Brussels sprouts	String beans (green and yellow)
Cabbage	Summer squash
Cauliflower	Tomatoes
Celery	Tomato juice
Eggplant	Turnips
Green pepper	Zucchini

Cooked greens: One exchange is ½ c. (125 mL) cooked.

Beet	Mustard
Chard	Spinach
Dandelion	Turnip

The following vegetables, eaten raw, may be used as desired.

Bean sprouts	Cucumbers	Parsley
Cauliflower	Endive	Radishes
Celery	Escarole	Watercress
Chicory	Lettuce	
Chinese cabbage	Mushrooms	

Starchy vegetables are on the Bread Exchange.

Fruit Exchange

Fruit and juices should not contain sugar. Sugar substitutes may be added, if desired. One exchange contains 10 grams carbohydrates and 40 calories.

Apples	1 small
Applesauce	½ c. (125 mL)
Apricots	2 medium
Banana	½ small
Berries	
Blackberries	½ c. (125 mL)
Blueberries	½ c. (125 mL)
Cherries	10 large
Raspberries	½ c. (125 mL)
Strawberries	¾ c. (190 mL)
Citrus Fruits	
Grapefruit	½ small
Lemon	as desired
Lime	as desired
Orange	1 small
Nectarine	1 medium
Tangerine	1 medium
Cranberries	as desired
Dried Fruits	
Apples	2 halves

Apricots	4 halves
Figs	1
Peaches	2 halves
Pears	2 halves
Prunes	2 medium
Raisins	2 T. (30 mL)
Grapes	12
Juices	
Apple juice or cider	⅓ c. (90 mL)
Cranberry (no sugar)	as desired
Grapefruit	½ c. (125 mL)
Grape	¼ c. (60 mL)
Orange	½ c. (125 mL)
Pineapple	⅓ c. (90 mL)
Prune	¼ c. (60 mL)
Tangerine	½ c. (125 mL)
Peach	1 medium
Pear	1 medium
Pineapple	½ c. (125 mL)
Plums	2 medium

Bread Exchange

One exchange contains 15 grams carbohydrate, 2 grams protein and 70 calories.

Bagel	½ small
Bread	
White (including French and Italian)	1 slice
Whole or cracked wheat	1 slice
Rye or pumpernickel	1 slice
Raisin	1 slice
Party rye	3 small rounds
Pita	¼ slice
Thin slice (white or dark)	1½ slices
Hollywood	2 slices
Cornbread, 2-in. (5-cm) square; omit 1 fat exchange	1 slice
Boston brown 3 × ½ in. (8 × 1 cm)	1 slice
Dinner roll	1 small
English muffin	½ small

Plain muffin; omit 1 fat exchange	1
Biscuit, 2 in. (5 cm); omit 1 fat exchange	1
Sandwich roll or bun	1
Bread croutons	1 c. (250 mL)
Bread stick, 8 × ½ in. (20 × 1½ cm)	2
Bread stick, 4 × ¼ in. (10 cm × 5 mm)	6
Tortilla or taco shell, 6 in. (15 cm)	3
Bread crumbs (fine)	¼ c. (60 mL)
Gingerbread, 2 in. (5 cm); omit 1 fat exchange	1
Bread stuffing; omit 1 fat exchange	½ c. (125 mL)
Toast, melba	4 oblong, or 8 round
Cake, pound, 3 × 3 × ½ in. (8 × 8 × 1 cm); omit 1 fat exchange	1
Cake, sponge or angel food, 1½ in. (4 cm) cube	1
Cereal	
Bran or bran buds	¼ c. (60 mL)
Bran flakes	½ c. (125 mL)
Unsweetened cereal	¾ c. (180 mL)
Unsweetened puff cereal	1 c. (250 mL)
Cooked cereals	½ c. (125 mL)
Chinese noodles	½ c. (125 mL)
Cookies	
Vanilla wafers	5
Gingersnaps	5
Lorna Doone shortbread	3
Fig Newtons, ½ oz. (15 g)	1
Plain, 3 in. (8 cm)	1
Oreo sandwich; omit 1 fat exchange	2
Crackers	
Animal	8
Arrowroot	3
Bugles; omit 2 fat exchanges	30
Doo Dads; omit 1 fat exchange	¾ c. (180 mL)
Holland rusks	2
Graham, 2½-in. (7-cm) square	2
Multishaped; omit 1 fat exchange	11
Matzo, 4 × 6 in. (10 × 15 cm)	½
Ritz, Hi Ho, etc.	6 rounds

Onion-flavored; omit 1 fat exchange	10
Oyster	20
Cheese Nips tidbits	60
Cheese; omit 1 fat exchange	6 rounds
RyKrisp	3
Shredded wheat wafers	3
Thin triangle; omit 1 fat exchange	14
Saltines, 2-in. (5-cm) square	5
Triscuit	5
Wheat Thins	10
Whistles; omit 1 fat exchange	30
Cream puff shell: omit 1 fat exchange	1 small
Doughnut, plain; omit 2 fat exchanges	1
Ice Cream	
Chocolate; omit 2 fat exchanges	½ c. (125 mL)
Vanilla; omit 2 fat exchanges	½ c. (125 mL)
Strawberry; omit 2 fat exchanges	½ c. (125 mL)
Dairy Queen; omit 1 fat exchange	⅓ c. (90 mL)
Marshmallows	3 large
Popcorn (unbuttered)	1 c. (250 mL)
Pretzels	20 thin, or 6 twists
Vegetables	
Dried beans, peas, lentils	½ c. (125 mL)
Corn	⅓ c. (90 mL)
Corn on the cob	1 small
Beets	½ c. (125 mL)
Carrots	½ c. (125 mL)
Onions	½ c. (125 mL)
Peas	½ c. (125 mL)
Potato	1 small
Potato chips; omit 2 fat exchanges	15, or 1 oz. (30 g) bag
Potatoes, shoestring; omit 2 fat exchanges	⅔ c. (180 g)
Pumpkin	1 c. (250 mL)
Rutabaga	½ c. (125 mL)
Tomato sauce	½ c. (125 mL)
Tomato paste	¼ c. (60 mL)
Winter squash	½ c. (125 mL)
Waffle, 4-in. (10-cm) square; omit 1 fat exchange	1
Zwieback	3

Meat Exchange

Lean Meat: One exchange contains 7 grams protein, 3 grams fat, and 55 calories.

Beef: chipped beef, chuck, flank, round and tenderloin steaks, all cuts rump and sirloin	1 oz. (30 g)
Lamb: any lean, trimmed cut	1 oz. (30 g)
Veal: any lean, trimmed cut	1 oz. (30 g)
Poultry (without skin): chicken, turkey, Cornish hen, pheasant	1 oz. (30 g)
Fish and seafood: any fresh or frozen	1 oz. (30 g)
Canned fish or seafood: packed in water	¼ c. (60 mL)

Medium-fat meat: One exchange contains 7 grams protein, 5 grams fat, and 75 calories.

Beef: ground beef (15% fat)	1 oz. (30 g)
Pork: loin shoulder and leg cuts, ham, Canadian bacon, Boston butt	1 oz. (30 g)
Egg	1
Cheese: white	1 oz. (30 g)
Cottage cheese	¼ c. (60 mL)

High-fat meat: One exchange contains 7 grams protein, 8 grams fat, and 100 calories.

Beef: ground beef (20% fat), brisket, rib and club cuts	1 oz. (30 g)
Pork: ground pork, rib cuts	1 oz. (30 g)
Poultry: duck, goose, capons	1 oz. (30 g)
Cheese: cheddar type	1 oz. (30 g)
Cold cuts and wieners	1

Fat Exchange

One exchange contains 5 grams fat and 45 calories.

Margarine or butter	1 t. (5 mL)
Bacon, crisp	1 slice
Cream, light (20%)	2 T. (30 mL)
heavy (40%)	1 T. (15 mL)
sour	2 T. (30 mL)
Mayonnaise	1 t. (5 mL)
Oil, cooking	1 t. (5 mL)
Gravy	2 T. (30 mL)
Nuts	
Almonds	10 whole
Brazil	2 whole
Cashews	5 whole
Peanuts	12 whole
Pecans	6 halves
Walnuts	6 halves
Olives	5 small
Tartar sauce	2 t. (10 mL)
Whipped cream	2 T. (30 mL)

Note: If diet requires only polyunsaturated fats, consult your doctor or diet counsellor.

Nutritional Information of Product Labels

Food manufacturers now label their products with nutritional information. This information can be very useful to anyone using the American Diabetes Association's exchange list in their diets. The labels give the number of calories and the grams of protein, carbohydrates and fat in each serving. Most often they are listed as in the example below:

NUTRITIONAL INFORMATION PER SERVING
Servings per container: 12
Serving Size (Cookie): 3
Calories per serving: 170
Protein: 2 g
Carbohydrates: 22 g
Fat: 7 g

With this information you can work out the food exchange on any product. The exchange list below is needed for calculations.

EXCHANGE	CALORIES	CARBO-HYDRATE (grams)	PROTEIN (grams)	FAT (grams)
Milk				
Whole	170	12	8	10
2%	125	12	8	5
Skim	80	12	8	0
Vegetable	36	7	2	0
Fruit	40	10	0	0
Bread	68	15	2	0
Meat				
Lean	55	0	7	3
Medium fat	78	0	7	6
High fat	100	0	7	8
Fat	45	0	0	5

Compare the nutrient value on the label with the nutrient values on the exchange list. Count whole and nearest half exchanges.

	Exchange	C	P	F
1. List the grams of carbohydrates, protein and fat per serving.		22	2	7
2. Subtract carbohydrates first. Bread exchange has 15 carbohydrates + 2 protein.	1 bread	−15	−2	
		7	0	7
3. Compare the next nearest carbohydrate exchange. Fruit exchange has 10.	1 fruit	−10		
		0	0	7
4. Compare fat exchange	1 fat			−5
		0	0	2

You have 2 grams of fat left—or approximately ½ fat exchange; therefore, your exchange on 1 serving of this product is equivalent to 1 bread, 1 fruit, 1½ fat.

5. Check with calories
    1 bread =   68 calories
    1 fruit   =   40 calories
    1½ fat   =   67 calories
                    175   (Product information states 170.)

Most exchanges figured on foods are not exact.

Selected Bibliography

American Diabetes Association. "American Diabetes Association Issues Statement on Aspartame in Diet Soft Drinks and Foods." News from American Diabetes Association, Inc. (Oct., 1983).

Chase, H. Peter. "Diabetes and Diet." *Food Technology* (Dec., 1979).

Crapo, Phyllis A. and Jerrold M. Olefsky. "Food Fallacies and Blood Sugar." *The New England Journal of Medicine* (July 7, 1983).

Crapo, Phyllis A. and Jerrold M. Olefsky, "Fructose—Its Characteristics, Physiology, and Metabolism." *Nutrition Today* (July–Aug., 1980).

Crapo, Phyllis A. and Margaret A. Powers. "Alias: Sugar." *Diabetes Forecast* (1981).

Diabetes Dateline. "FDA Approves Aspartame as Low-Calorie Sweetener." Department of Health and Human Services (July–Aug., 1981).

Dwivedi, Basant K. ed. *Low-Calorie and Special Dietary Foods.* The Chemical Rubber Co. (1978): 61–73.

Franz, Marion. "Is Aspartame Safe?" *Diabetes Forecast* (May–June, 1984).

Kimura, K.K. "Dietary Sugars in Health and Disease." Life Sciences Research Office (Oct., 1976).

Koivisto, Veikko A. "Fructose as a Dietary Sweetener in Diabetes Mellitus." *Diabetes Care,* Vol. 1, No. 4 (July–Aug., 1978).

Olefsky, Jerrold and Phyllis Crapo. "Fructose, Xylitol, and Sorbitol." *Diabetes Care,* Vol. 3, No. 2 (March–April, 1980).

Tolbot, John M. and Kenneth D. Fisher. "The Need for Special Foods and Sugar Substitutes by Individuals with Diabetes Mellitus." *Diabetes Care,* Vol. 1 (July–Aug., 1978).

Public Health Service Food and Drug Administration. Department of Health and Human Services. "Aspartame: Commissioner's Final Decision." Part IV, Federal Register, Vol. 46, No. 142 (July 24, 1981): 38283–38308.

Index

155